610.72
RESEARCH SKILLS & TECHNIQUES

NURSING AND HEALTH-CARE RESEARCH

A Practical Guide

WY
20·5
COJ

Mine

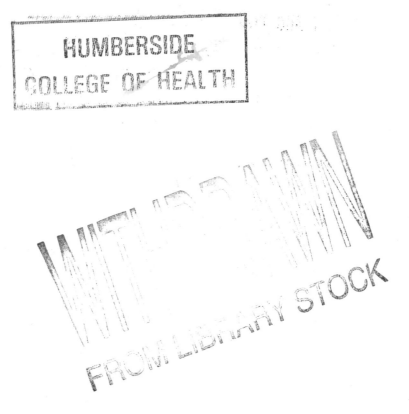

NURSING AND HEALTH-CARE RESEARCH

A Practical Guide

The Use and Application of Research for Nurses and Other Health Care Professionals

WENDY COUCHMAN MSc BA CSS
*Senior Lecturer, Department of Nursing and Social Service
Dorset Institute
Poole*

JANE DAWSON MSc SRN HV
*Research and Development Project Officer,
Portsmouth District Health Authority*

SCUTARI PRESS
London

© Scutari Press 1990

A division of Scutari Projects, the publishing company of
the Royal College of Nursing

First published 1990
Reprinted 1992

British Library Cataloguing in Publication Data

Couchman, Wendy
  Nursing and health-care research.
  1. Medicine. Nursing. Research
  I. Title   II. Dawson, Jane
  610.73'072

  ISBN 1–871364–22–1

Typeset by Columns of Reading
Printed and bound in Great Britain by
Biddles Ltd, Guildford and King's Lynn

Contents

To our families for
their patience
and our colleagues for
their support

Preface

'Research' is one of those words guaranteed to send a *frisson* of fear through the novice! What this book tries to do is show that research is really quite a 'friendly', everyday activity. It is hard work sometimes, but satisfying and straightforward if you follow a systematic, problem-solving approach.

Why is it important for nurses to know about research? Since the Briggs Report (Committee on Nursing, 1972, Cmnd 5115, HMSO) nurses have been urged to keep up to date with research, and there has been a lot of emphasis in policy statements on nursing as a research-based profession. Every profession needs to develop a body of knowledge, in fact, so that individuals do not proceed by trial and error, each 're-inventing the wheel'.

Nurses can use and build on the work of others to improve practice and the service to patients or clients. With the current emphasis upon quality assurance and accountability, it is also important for nurses to be able to evaluate and justify their practice.

Our book has two aims: first, to help to close the gap between what is known and what is done in nursing practice by giving enough familiarity with the research process to understand and evaluate relevant research findings; and second, to develop skills so that individuals can design and implement small-scale research projects that critically examine their own work.

The book, therefore, operates at the two levels of research appreciation and beginning actual research. It is essentially a self-instruction guide to research methods. Practical exercises and activities are suggested in each chapter to promote the relevant skills for a research project. A range of quantitative and qualitative methods are discussed as options to solve research problems.

We have also used throughout a fictitious nursing research project, on a topical subject, to illustrate the steps and the snags. In it we consider the decisions that a team of nurses in hospital and in the community must make in investigating the implications of a proposed change in policy. Following the stages in the project helps to capture the logic and the excitement of research. Each chapter develops the themes of the project to the next stage, from the origins of the idea, through the research design, to the analysis and communication of results.

A variety of textbooks on research methodology has become available in this country and from the United States to cater for a growing interest and need in nursing. Many are based on a step-by-step approach or describe exemplars in nursing research. This is, however, the first text designed as a complete introductory workbook, combined with the use of an extended exemplar to give the essential details of research in a lively, relevant way.

The book, therefore, has a wide potential audience. Individual nurses and midwives of all grades and specialities can use it for updating and professional development as recommended by current policies. The workbook approach should be helpful to tutors teaching groups from basic to postbasic levels of education, where 'research awareness' is now part of the curriculum and may involve some project work. The exercises in each chapter can be adapted for both individual and group work. The book can also serve as a foundation for more formal research training such as that provided by the ENB course No. 870, degree and diploma courses and research degrees. Although aimed mainly at nurses, it will also be of interest to allied caring professionals such as paramedics, therapists, health educators and social workers, who are similarly interested in research.

Both of the authors have successfully tried this 'learning by doing' approach in teaching research methods on a wide range of nursing and community courses, from short course to degree level. Wendy Couchman is a Senior Lecturer in Research Methods and Behavioural Sciences in the Department of Nursing and Social Service, Dorset Institute of Higher Education; Jane Dawson is Research and Development Project Officer for Portsmouth District Health Authority. They are also both involved in research projects in the health and social services. Jane Dawson's areas of interest are the effects of day surgery and early discharge on community nursing, and a comparison of methods of assessing manpower requirements in a district nursing service. Her current research is on quality assurance in general nursing and midwifery. Wendy Couchman has been involved in several surveys on the professional development of nurses, and projects on services for ESMI patients and adults with mental handicap. Currently, she is studying day services for adults with multiple handicaps.

WENDY COUCHMAN
JANE DAWSON
1989

1

Research in Nursing

Hightown General Hospital

At a meeting of the staff on Ward 4, a 24-bed surgical ward, Student Nurse Green raises the question of ward-based research projects. She is currently studying research methods as part of her training. Her suggestion is met with a variety of responses.

Research seems a rather remote activity to some of the group. Quite a few have had some experience of taking part in projects for managers, tutors or academic research teams but have never thought of initiating their own research. Some people feel pessimistic about having the power to make any changes. One cynic says that nursing research is done by 'failed practitioners' so how can it be relevant to her practice! Others react rather guiltily because they know nurses are now expected to be involved in research, and they would like to be, but don't really know how to go about it.

'It's all very well expecting us to do research like the medical profession', says one of the staff, 'but they have study days and support systems. With all the pressures at work it's difficult for us to get free time, so where do we fit in research?'

Some important questions are being raised here – and in nursing everywhere. We will use this fictitious situation, and how it evolves, throughout the book to make our discussion of the research process more 'real'.

DEFINING RESEARCH

Student Nurse Green could have pointed out that they were all using research skills already. If research is defined as:

'An attempt to extend knowledge through systematic, scientific enquiry' (Hockey, 1986)

1

then most nurses have the necessary skills. They follow similar systematic procedures as part of the nursing process with individual patients. They use methods like those in research to find new solutions in the management of their work.

Scientific enquiry is really a problem-solving model, the application of some basic skills in a series of logical steps:

1. A problem is stated.
2. An hypothesis is formulated for testing (i.e. a possible explanation is suggested).
3. Facts are gathered from observation or experimentation.
4. These facts are interpreted to see if the hypothesis was right.
5. Conclusions are drawn about solutions to the problem.

For centuries the scientific approach has been regarded as the finest way to establish new knowledge. Certainly, in nursing research it has been found more consistent as a means of finding out facts than the alternatives offered by tradition, authority or trial and error. This applies not only to finding out new knowledge, but also to checking existing knowledge through replication studies. Nursing needs to base practice with patients on very sound evidence if it is to develop as a discipline.

The principles of systematic research and the debate between different methods and degrees of scientific rigour will be discussed more fully in Chapter 5 on research design.

SUPPORT FOR RESEARCH

Some nurses make a personal choice to devote some of their own time to research projects to enhance their career and professional development. It is sometimes possible to get study time for research through district or regional scholarships or, if the research is pursued as part of a research diploma or degree, at a higher education establishment. This also provides guidance if there is no expertise locally. It is still worth looking for local help. There are more graduate nurses with research experience around now and some districts are appointing research nurses. Try enquiring at the school of nursing. Help may also be available in other disciplines such as medicine and psychology.

In our scenario, Staff Nurse Baker, who is studying for a diploma in nursing course, knows of a tutor at the School of Nursing with a research background. After some more discussion at the meeting, it is agreed that Staff Nurse Baker should approach the tutor and ask if she could come and talk to the staff team about research in nursing.

INFLUENCING CHANGE

When the tutor does visit at the next meeting, she explains that if nurses become involved in investigating their own practice, this should help to overcome the argument that nursing research is irrelevant. Even if the research is done by outsiders, the practitioner should have enough understanding to participate, to help to define and resolve the real problems.

Nurses need to understand better why they do what they do. Many practices persist because 'they have always been done this way'. An example is the practice of salt baths for healing wounds. When subjected to research scrutiny, however, such practices are found to have no real benefit, and are wasteful of time and effort.

Nurses may also need to provide data to justify their practice to others. In the increasingly political and economic arena of health care today, evidence is needed on the effectiveness of services. Practitioners must enter into a dialogue on what is to be measured, and how, rather than leaving measurement to others who may not take account of the important factors.

There are numerous cases where nurses have been able to effect changes in practice through research. A good example is Jean Moores' study of the treatment of leg ulcers in the community (Moores, 1987).

Nurses who feel powerless to influence change should perhaps look at the history of changes in policy. Many of these have followed from grass-roots action. Decisions are not made by management alone. Change can, therefore, be initiated both 'top down' and 'bottom up' – what has been called 'the shower and bidet principle'!

USING RESEARCH

The tutor reminds the group that, according to the Briggs Report (Committee on Nursing, 1972), *using* research is just as important as *doing* it. There is now a wealth of knowledge from nursing research started by the classic RCN studies of the 1960s and 1970s. There is still a gap, however, between what is known and what is done. The findings of the classic studies in many cases have not been put into practice on the ward, nor have they yet found their way into all nurse training syllabuses. Despite the findings of Hamilton-Smith in *Nil by Mouth?* (1972), for example, that lengthy preoperative fasting could not be justified for all patients, this practice still persists on a national scale.

Jennifer Hunt (1984a) lists four main reasons why nurses do not use research findings:

1. *Lack of knowledge.* Nurses simply have not heard about relevant research, have poor access to libraries or do not know how to evaluate and apply the findings.
2. *Disbelief.* Nurses remain unconvinced by data that challenge traditional practice.
3. *Lack of permission.* Nurses may not be allowed to challenge traditional practice by introducing change suggested by research.

4. *Lack of incentive.* Nurses are not rewarded for introducing change by positive feedback or by financial or status incentives.

Hunt argues that research must become integral to practice and rewards must be provided.

PROFESSIONALISM

Staff Nurse Baker adds a relevant point from her current studies: that the increasing emphasis on research is consistent with the growth of the profession. Sociologists have shown (Schröck, 1987) that the transition of an occupation such as nursing to the status of a profession is characterised by elements such as:

1. The length of training being increased.
2. Assessment and examinations becoming more rigorous as the means of qualification.
3. More focus on research to establish a unique body of knowledge or theory.

There is evidence of all these changes in nursing today, confirmed by reports such as Project 2000.

STRUCTURE OF THE BOOK

This book has been structured around the steps in the research process that you follow whether you are doing a research project or reading about one. This will be demonstrated in each chapter by examples from our scenario, and through exercises to develop research skills.

You will see that the series of steps in research follows the same logical process as the scientific approach outlined earlier:

1. Stating research problem or questions.
2. Reviewing relevant literature.
3. Choosing research design.
4. Collecting data.
5. Analysing data.
6. Discussing results.
7. Reporting results.

The process is, in fact, more *cyclic* (Figure 1.1) because there may be several points in a study where the researcher either refers back to an earlier step or repeats certain steps to refine the design. A completed study also raises questions to be pursued in other research.

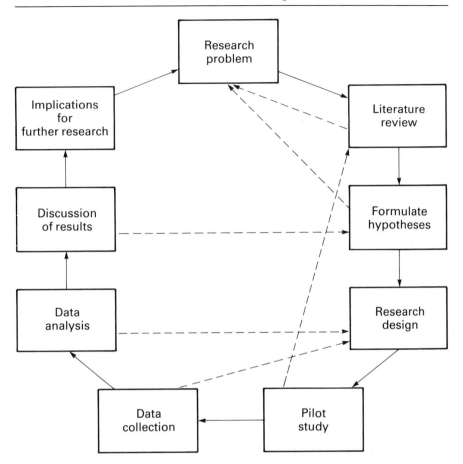

Figure 1.1 The research cycle

GUIDE TO READING

The book has been written sequentially so that, like Alice, you can start at the beginning and go on until you reach the end. If you are only interested in one topic at a time, each chapter does make sense when read separately.

The early stages of choosing and reading around a research topic are covered in Chapters 2 and 3. Chapter 4 deals with step-by-step techniques for reading research critically. Chapter 5 addresses the issues at the research design stage. Chapters 6 to 8 present a range of different research styles. Chapter 9 raises associated matters such as ethics.

The final steps in the research process are discussed in the last few chapters of the book. Chapter 10 is on the analysis of data and its presentation, Chapter 11 deals with different media for the communication and publication of research findings, and support for research is covered in Chapter 12.

Note

The feminine pronoun 'she' will be used throughout in the generic sense to mean 'he' or 'she'.

BIBLIOGRAPHY

Committee on Nursing (1972) *Report of the Committee on Nursing* (Chairman Prof. A Briggs). Cmnd. 5115, London: HMSO.

Cormack D F S (ed.) (1984) *The Research Process in Nursing*, Part I. Oxford: Blackwell.

Hamilton-Smith S C (1972) *Nil by Mouth?* London: Royal College of Nursing.

Hockey L (1985) *Nursing Research: Mistakes and Misconceptions*. Edinburgh: Churchill Livingstone.

Hockey L (1986) Nursing research: its pleasures, problems and potential for nursing. Paper presented at Wessex Regional Research Conference at Dorset Institute of Higher Education, Poole, 29 November 1986.

Hunt J (1984a) Why don't we use these findings? *Nursing Mirror,* **158** (8): 29.

Hunt J (1984b) Step by Step. *Nursing Mirror,* **158** (1): 29–30.

McFarlane J (1980) Nursing as a research-based profession. *Nursing Times,* **76** (13).

Milne A (1981) Hitches, hurdles and hopes. *Nursing Mirror,* **152** (2): 30–32.

Moores J (1987) The nurse v. leg ulcers. *Journal of District Nursing,* **5** (9): 16–21.

Polit D and Hungler B (1983) *Nursing Research: Principles and Methods*, Chs. 1 and 3. Philadelphia: J B Lippincott.

Schröck R A (1987) Professionalisation – a critical examination. *Recent Advances in Nursing,* **18**: 12–24.

Treece E W and Treece J W (1977) *Elements of Research in Nursing*. New York: Mosby.

2

Making a Start in Research

True research is not simply a matter of gathering information. It is finding answers to questions or solutions to problems. So the first step in research is choosing or defining your problem.

In order to illustrate this early stage in research, let's revisit the team on Ward 4.

SCENARIO

In an attempt to reduce surgical waiting lists, hospital management are considering introducing day surgery and five-day stay to Ward 4. Some of the staff on the ward who are interested in research agree to use these changes as a research problem for investigation.

The sister of the ward, Sister Jones, realises that the changes will radically affect the operation of the ward, but is unsure as to the nature of these effects.

Staff Nurse Baker is concerned that the new plan will interfere with the ward's commitment to the use of the nursing process.

Student Nurse Green sees an opportunity for a small project for an assignment for her course.

The community nurse, Sister Brown, whose liaison with the ward is good, can tell that the changes will affect her work-load, but does not know to what extent.

Each member of the team, therefore, has a slightly different approach to the problem.

FINDING IDEAS

The approach taken by each of our team will be used as themes for the following chapters, demonstrating a range of research methods. We will return to a discussion of how the team tackled their problems after some guidelines and exercises to develop your own research skills in starting projects. Most of the exercises can be done individually or in group work.

Some of the best nursing research ideas were inspired by problems in everyday practice that niggle or puzzle, such as our example. Some of the best nursing research is, therefore, done by practitioners, rather than outside researchers, because they are often in the best position to judge what are the important factors. We would also argue that the practitioner is in an ideal position for communicating and implementing ideas from the research. A systematic research attitude will in turn inform practice. The ability to be objective is of course vital.

Simply stated, both the researcher and the nurse continually need to question practice, and challenge taken-for-granted assumptions in the same way as they did on the first day in the job. Ideas for research projects can also be generated through reading and study, as we will see from the exercise later.

Unfortunately, finding research ideas is a difficult and uncomfortable process, accompanied by feelings of vagueness, aimlessness and indecision. It can be reassuring to recognise that this is a necessary state in the evolution of any creative activity. Even Einstein must have gone through the agonising process to reach his brilliant 'hunches'!

Although it is a creative process, there are ways of introducing structure to minimise the pain and maximise opportunities for ideas, which we will show through some exercises. Most of these are based on the simple problem-solving model:

1. Define the problem.
2. Generate possible solutions.
3. Select and implement the best solution.
4. Evaluate the outcome.

Thinkers like Edward de Bono (1970) promote the positive value of spending time at this stage to explore a problem fully, through lateral thinking and brainstorming. It is, therefore, wise to relax and not rush in order to make the right choices, or choices that you won't regret later.

Practise your brainstorming skills with this exercise:

Exercise

Stage 1

Imagine that you have been cast ashore on a desert island naked, with nothing but a belt! What could you do with the belt?

Rules

1. Think of as many ideas as possible – spend at least 5 minutes on this stage.
2. Aim for quantity not quality at this point – keep an open mind.
3. Don't spend too long on each idea – keep them bubbling.

4. Do not criticise or dismiss any suggestions yet.
5. Write everything down, however nonsensical or outrageous it seems – apparently silly or irrelevant ideas can often lead to a new way of looking at a problem.
6. Build on or combine ideas to make new ones.

Stage 2

When the ideas begin to dry up, look again at your list. Now you can be critical and evaluative. Which seems the most feasible? Can you combine elements of several ideas?

Can you see that you are likely to have come up with a better solution than if you had taken the first idea that occurred to you, which is the usual 'vertical' thinking or logic?

Discussion

Obviously there are no right answers with this approach. People who do the exercise become very imaginative with possibilities for using the belt in different ways – ranging from as a source of food, through various tools, utensils and weapons, to a means of ending it all! They usually end up with an optimum combination of uses.

Now try brainstorming a list of researchable ideas in your field of nursing:

Exercise

Where do research problems come from?

Use the headings below as prompts to jot down ideas and questions. These three areas are the main sources for research topics in nursing:

Experience (the most common source of ideas)
Things that are puzzling, problematic or challenging in everyday practice (e.g. instruction on use of medication on discharge from hospital, effective communication between professionals).

Questions to ask:

- Why do we do this . . .?
- Why this way . . .?
- Who's it for . . .?
- What if . . .?

Reading
Ideas that arise from relevant literature: gaps left in research; need for replication; recommendations for research from other studies; contributions

to a current issue or debate in the professional journals (e.g. the nursing process, treatment of pressure sores).

Questions to ask:

- Would that work here . . .?
- What next . . .?

Theory

Translating and testing theoretical concepts in the real world (e.g. nursing models, communication theories). Adding to the body of nursing knowledge.

Questions to ask:

- What does that mean in practice . . .?
- Can that be proved . . .?

Discussion

In practice you would spend some time exploring ideas, sounding out colleagues, family and friends – providing they are prepared to follow the rules of brainstorming and suspend all criticism at this stage! Ideally you would find a mentor with whom to discuss your ideas and the project as it progressed. This could be a colleague, a manager, a tutor. Gradually you would need to begin sorting and prioritising your list of potential research projects to narrow the focus, to select the most feasible.

CHOOSING A TOPIC

Here is a check-list of questions to help you choose more critically the most feasible topic from your list:

Exercise

How do I choose?

Ask these questions of each of the possible topics on your list to decide which is the most researchable. You may find it helpful to work through the questions and the list with other people:

Is it really a problem?
- Is it only me who sees it as a problem?
- Who else finds it a problem?

Is it a significant problem?
- Is it important?

- Is it too trivial?
- Will it benefit anyone?
- Will it be useful?
- Will it increase knowledge?
- Will it check assumptions?
- Will it inform policy or practice?

Is it a researchable problem?
- Is it morally, ethically or politically dubious?
- Do I need permission from the ethical committee?
- Is it too philosophical?
- Can it be precisely defined and measured?
- Do I have the necessary knowledge and skills?

How feasible is it?
- Is there time?
- Are people available?
- Will they consent and co-operate?
- What facilities and equipment are needed?
- How much will it cost?
- Do I have financial support?
- Is it worth it?
- Is it familiar?

Is it interesting?
- Is it newsworthy?
- Will anyone care?
- Do I care enough?

Discussion

All of these questions represent important considerations, not least the last. It is vital that one is excited and made curious by the topic from the outset in order to be sustained through the 'dark days' when things go wrong, or in the middle of a project when you seem a long way from the beginning and a long way from the end. You need to 'own' the project, and beware of being persuaded to follow someone else's idea or 'hobby horse' – it will be difficult to stay motivated.

RESEARCH STATEMENTS

A check-list helps the beginning researcher to reach a decision on the broad topic. The next stage is to refine the topic to a written, formal statement of the problem or question to be answered by the research design. This clarifies thinking and involves some detailed planning of specific areas of interest. If you can get this right at the start, the project will be much easier to follow and achieve.

For example, the topic 'nurse–patient interaction' is too broad and likely to lead the researcher up many interesting avenues, which go nowhere in particular. The topic is open to so many interpretations, all potentially researchable if the terms are defined more precisely, as follows:

Broad topic

- Nurse–patient interaction.

Researchable topics

- The importance of touch in communication with elderly patients.
- Asking questions of women in labour.
- The teaching of counselling skills to student nurses.
- Giving information to children before an operation.
- Social skills training with psychiatric patients.
- Instructions to heart patients leaving hospital.
- Telephone links with at-risk patients in the community.

Writing research statements is, of course, similar to writing objectives in the nursing process, and the same general principles apply: the communication of clear, concrete and unambiguous statements of intent. In other words you avoid 'fuzzies'! Robert Mager who has written several instructional and entertaining books about goal setting and objective writing has a cautionary tale about 'fuzzies':

Extract from *Goal Analysis* by Robert F Mager (1974)

Once upon a time in the land of Fuzz, King Aling called in his cousin Ding and commanded, 'Go ye out into all of Fuzzland and find me the goodest of men, whom I shall reward for his goodness'.

'But how will I know one when I see one?' asked the Fuzzy.

'Why, he will be *sincere*', scoffed the king, and whacked off a leg for his impertinence.

So, the Fuzzy limped out to find a good man. But soon he returned, confused and empty-handed.

'But how will I know one when I see one?' he asked again.

'Why, he will be *dedicated*', grumbled the king, and whacked off another leg for his impertinence.

So the Fuzzy hobbled away once more to look for the goodest of men. But again he returned, confused and empty-handed.

'But how will I know one when I see one?', he pleaded.

'Why, he will have *internalised his growing awareness*', fumed the king, and whacked off another leg for for his impertinence.

So the Fuzzy, now on his last leg, hopped out to continue his search. In time, he returned with the most sincere and dedicated Fuzzy in all of Fuzzland, and stood him before the king.

'Why this man won't do at all', roared the king. 'He is much too thin to suit me'. Whereupon, he whacked off the last leg of the Fuzzy, who fell to the floor with a squishy thump.

The moral of this fable is that . . . *if you can't tell one when you see one, you may wind up without a leg to stand on.*

There is a picture of a 'fuzzy' in Figure 2.1, which we will define as: 'a vague, ambiguous and often abstract statement of intent'.

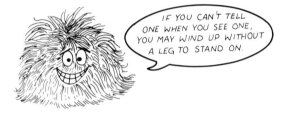

Figure 2.1   A 'fuzzy'

Try spotting the 'fuzzies' in the following statements:

Exercise

Which of the following research statements are fuzzy?

1. Looking at hospital visitors.
2. The effects of reorganisation on the ward sister's role.
3. Interaction between professionals in the psychiatric community team.
4. Use of the nursing process.
5. District nurses' rating of stress factors in their work-load.
6. Confidentiality of patient records.

Discussion

Statements 1, 4 and 6 are fuzzy, 2, 3 and 5 are non-fuzzy.

The test is, it is a fuzzy if it is difficult to know exactly what the researcher intends, or the statement is open to misinterpretation. As a further exercise you could try restating the fuzzies in non-fuzzy terms, relevant to your own field.

In the hunt for fuzzies in research statements, you can also apply the 'Hey Dad' test. If Dad would have difficulty in seeing what you mean, then it is a fuzzy. For instance, what exactly would he see if you said you were studying nurse–patient interaction or hospital visitors?

Fuzzy words are vague abstractions ('being' words), whereas non-fuzzy words suggest performance ('doing' words).

The 'Hey Dad' Test

Hey Dad! Come and see me . . .

Fuzzies	Non-fuzzies
knowing	comparing
understanding	contrasting
appreciating	constructing
believing	identifying
developing	defining
internalising	discriminating
enjoying	sorting

Sometimes it is difficult to express intentions fully in non-fuzzy performance terms, and in these cases you need to describe how you are going to indicate or measure the abstract quality. If, for example, you were interested in attitudes about a particular subject, you need to consider the means of assessing these – whether by interview, or rating scale or some other method.

The refinement of research statements is a continuing process until a formal written statement of the problem is reached. This should cover 'who does what, where, when and how'. The statement must also specify outcome and not just the process of the research – the 'ends' as well as the 'means'. To summarise, a research statement should spell out detail explicitly, so that anyone could read it and have a good idea what the researcher was intending to do.

This little poem, also based on Mager's work (1968), says it all:

There once was a nurse
Who always scored first
And won fame and acclaim if not pay.
  Achievements by millions
  Or possibly zillions
  Surrounded her all of the day

When finally asked
How she managed her tasks
By the boss who wanted to know,
  'Now listen!' she cried,

Three fingers held high,
If the way you want me to show.

'To rise from a zero
To Big Nursing Hero,
To answer these questions you'll strive:
Where am I going,
How shall I get there, and
How will I know I've arrived?'

The moral is then, if you don't know where you're going, how can you tell when you've got there?

Figure 2.2 is an illustration of how our example of nurse–patient interaction could be translated into a workable research statement by successive steps.

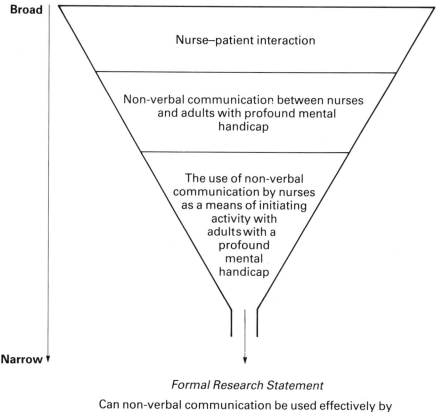

Broad

Nurse–patient interaction

Non-verbal communication between nurses and adults with profound mental handicap

The use of non-verbal communication by nurses as a means of initiating activity with adults with a profound mental handicap

Narrow

Formal Research Statement

Can non-verbal communication be used effectively by nurses as a means of initiating leisure activities with adults with a profound mental handicap in a residential setting?

Figure 2.2 Translating a research problem into a research statement

It is sometimes easier to restate the topic as a question, as this seems to give a sense of urgency or drive to find the answer by the research process. Sometimes you might want to develop the research statement further to a hypothesis, but this would normally be after the literature search stage, and we will discuss hypotheses in a later chapter. Remember that you are not concerned, either, with how to answer the research question (i.e. the method) at this stage, otherwise the methodological tail tends to wag the dog. Do not assume yet, for instance, that you need to do a survey just because a lot of research seems to use that method. There may be other methods more appropriate as a means of answering your question.

Exercise

Try now to restate your research topic from the earlier exercise either as a statement or as a question. Add any explanatory notes that seem necessary.

Remember to plan and specify in as much detail as possible to communicate the ideas clearly.

Check carefully for fuzzies!

This is a useful exercise to do in a group.

We will return now to our fictitious research team to see how they tackled their problems. In the following chapters we will see how they then put ideas into practice, through the research process.

SCENARIO

At their meeting the members of the team affected by the proposed changes to surgery stays agreed that they already had their broad topic for a research project, which could be justified by its priority and importance to the everyday running of a service for patients. All involved had discussed the problems with colleagues and other professionals, such as the consultant. They decided to begin by brainstorming the issues involved, listing thoughts as they occurred on a large sheet of paper; and this is what their list looked like:

1. Work-load
   - ward
   - community (extra time?)
2. Present situation
   - which patients likely 1 day/5 day?
   - which longer stays?
   - how change nursing process – different models – how work for surgery?
   - patients views, feelings – new and traditional systems?

From this list it became clear that, by narrowing and defining the topic to a series of questions, each member of the team could take a different yet complementary angle on the problem, according to their individual interest.

The list of questions (checked for fuzzies!) was allocated to team members as follows:

1. What is the average length of stay at present for various types of operation on this ward? (Sister Jones)
2. Which operations will be 5-day stay, which will be a day, and which longer than 5 days? (Sister Jones)
3. How have similar wards adapted the nursing process to the new system? (Staff Nurse Baker)
4. How would a different model of the nursing process work on our ward? (Sister Nurse Baker)
5. How will the proposed changes affect patients on the ward? (Student Nurse Green)
6. How much time do visits to different types of patient take after discharge from hospital? (Sister Brown)
7. Will the new system mean longer visits to discharged patients? (Sister Brown)

The next step for the team will be to undertake a review of the relevant literature, and this will be discussed in the next chapter.

BIBLIOGRAPHY

Calnan J (1984) *Coping with Research, the Complete Guide for Beginners.* London: Heinemann Medical Books.
Cormack D F S (ed.) (1984) *The Research Process in Nursing,* ch. 6. Oxford: Blackwell.
Darling V H and Rogers J (1986) *Research for Practising Nurses,* ch. 2. Basingstoke: Macmillan.
de Bono E (1970) *Lateral Thinking: A Textbook of Creativity.* Harmondsworth: Penguin Books.
Mager R F (1968) *Developing Attitude Toward Learning.* California: Fearon Pitman Publishing.
Mager R F (1974) *Goal Analysis.* California: Pitman Learning.
Mager R F (1975) *Preparing Instructional Objectives.* California: Fearon Publishing.
Polit D and Hungler B (1983) *Nursing Research: Principles and Methods,* ch. 5. Philadelphia: J B Lippincott.
Sheehan J (1985) Research series 1: Starting the study. *Nursing Mirror,* **160** (18): 17–18.
Treece E W and Treece J W (1977) *Elements of Research in Nursing.* New York: Mosby.

3

Reviewing the Literature

Probably the one factor which will have most influence on the way you go about your research is the literature search. If you read any major research report, you will find that a large part of it is devoted to a review of the literature.

Why is this? Why does it matter so much? When, and how, should it be done?

The first point to make is that the literature search is not something that is done just once and then forgotten. It is almost a continuous process throughout a project, although concentrated and directed according to the stage reached in the research process. The main literature search, which is carried out at the beginning of a research project, will probably take about one-quarter to one-third of the total time available for the research to conduct. After that, the literature is consulted for specific reasons, to help the development of the research tools for example or to look for an explanatory theory after the data have been analysed.

PRELIMINARY SEARCH

When you start to think about a certain subject and how research might be carried out into it, a review of the literature is essential. The aim at this stage is to gain an overview of the subject, to 'read around' it. This stage is very general, but inevitably it will become focused as you begin to identify more clearly what it is you wish to do.

DIRECTED LITERATURE SEARCH

As the thinking about the subject becomes focused, the literature search is more directed and specific regarding certain points:

The research question

From a vague idea of a subject, which you wish to know more about, the literature can help to define the precise research question that it is intended to answer. It will also help in formulating an hypothesis if the research is of a design which requires this. An hypothesis is the 'next stage' from the statement of the problem that we talked about in Chapter 2. For example, the statement:

The effects of reorganisation on the ward sister's role.

would lead to the hypothesis:

Reorganisation will significantly affect the role of the ward sister.

The point about rephrasing the statement in this way is that it makes clear exactly what the research is intended to investigate. The hypothesis can be tested, the statement cannot.

Sometimes, research that is purely exploratory in nature does not require an hypothesis. If, for example, you were not sure whether the reorganisation would indeed affect the ward sister's role but simply wanted to see what happened, a clear statement would be sufficient. The literature search can help you decide whether you have a testable hypothesis or whether your research should be more descriptive in nature.

The research design

The decisions that have to be made on the most appropriate way of going about answering that research question, or testing the hypothesis, will be aided by reading about previous studies. Seeing how other people tackled the same or similar research questions will demonstrate the advantages and pitfalls in various types of research design.

The research tools

You may find during a literature search that someone has used a particular questionnaire, or other measurement technique, which you feel it would be appropriate to use or adapt. As long as you can justify the application of that tool in the study, there is no reason why you should not do so.

The research criteria

Reading how other researchers have defined the variables in previous studies will provide some ideas about the definitions you will use. A variable is a unit (person, event or characteristic) that can vary. Age is a variable, nursing qualifications and attendance at out-patients are all variables. If for example the research concerns non-attenders at out-patients' clinics, precisely what is meant by non-attenders? Anyone who misses just one appointment or people who attend some appointments but miss some? The literature search will help you decide where best to direct your efforts.

Theory

The thorny question of how and where theory fits into research can only be resolved by reference to the literature. Reading the work of others may bring to your attention theory relevant to the research topic that you decide to test out or apply in a different way. Equally you may come across theoretical ideas with which you disagree, but at least this will serve to sharpen up your own thinking. If you started out without a clear theoretical framework before the data were collected, the literature may give meaning and explanation to the findings through theory generated by previous work. Chapter 5 discusses the place of theory in research.

Another way to think about the literature search is:

1. Research that has been done by others on the same subject; and
2. Research that is related in some way but was in other areas. For example, if you were interested in the cause and effect of stress in nurses it would be useful to look at published material on stress in teachers or some other occupational groups.

PURPOSES OF THE LITERATURE SEARCH

The purpose of the literature search is then to:

1. Find out what other research has already been conducted on the topic, or a related topic.
2. Give ideas on the research design and methodology and tools which could be appropriately applied.
3. Aid in the definition of the variables in the intended research.
4. Consider the theoretical framework that will underpin the study.
5. Put the project into the context of the broader body of knowledge in the field.

The literature reviewed can be of two kinds, research and non-research. Research literature, as it implies, reports on specific projects or studies conducted according to research principles. Non-research literature covers the opinions, experiences and theories that have some bearing on the subject or that relate to it in some way.

HOW TO CARRY OUT A LITERATURE SEARCH

Hospitals and schools of nursing usually have very good libraries now, and this is the place to start. The one nearest to you will probably be linked to others in the health region and to the British Library. This means that the library will be able to borrow books and articles that it does not itself stock. There may be a charge for this service, however, so find out about this. If there are a university, polytechnic or college of further education within reach, then the range of literature available to you opens up enormously. Most such establishments have some form of link with the health district, so it is worth contacting the librarian to find out what arrangements there are for health authority employees to borrow from them. The local authority library is well worth investigating, and there are also specialist libraries that concentrate on particular fields of study. A list of some of these is given at the end of this chapter.

The first thing to do when embarking on a literature search is to write down a list of key words. This means the words that are central to the research topic. The best way to do this is to state the research problem as simply as possible, trying to reduce it to one or two sentences. If you look back at Chapter 2 on refining the research statement, the importance of this stage and the technique of how to do this is discussed more fully. Once you have your formal written statement, then pick out the words which are central to this statement.

Our ward team might list the following key words from the series of questions that they defined.

- Current length of stay (specific operations).
- Probable operations for day surgery/5-day wards.
- Use/evaluation of nursing process.
- Community work-load.

Can you think of any more?

Another way into the literature is to list the authors you happen to know have written on the subject, then look up their work.

When you start your search there are three main sources of information:

BIBLIOGRAPHIES

Bibliographies are lists of published material, such as books, articles and sometimes papers given at conferences. These are listed both by subject (where your key words come in) and by author. The author, title, place and date of publication are given.

ABSTRACTS

These are similar to bibliographies, but in addition a summary of the material is given also. The abstract may simply outline the subject of the paper, without the results, or it may include the main results. This is particularly useful as then you can decide whether a particular publication is relevant to your needs before searching it out or sending for it.

INDEXES

Again, material is listed both by subject and by author, but only articles are given, not books. Most indexes scan journals internationally for material to be included, so not all the references you find will be available in English, or they may be in journals that are not held by many libraries in this country.

Bibliographies are usually in the form of booklets. Indexes are much weightier in size and content! A list of bibliographies, abstracts and indexes is given at the end of this chapter.

This information is also held on microfiche. These are small acetate sheets, each of which holds a large number of entries, and which are read under a special viewer. The fiche are usually classified alphabetically by author and title, with a separate alphabetical set of subject fiche, though as a rule they are confined to books, not journals. Virtually every library has a microfiche these days, so they are worth investigating.

The main drawback with abstracts and indexes is that they take time to compile, so it may be 6 months after the date of publication before a paper is included in them. Indeed, because the cycle of research, presentation and publication as thesis, article and book, is such a painstaking and time-consuming affair, there can be an interval of 4 or 5 years beteween commencing the research and the final appearance in an abstract or index. Current awareness facilities, such as the Health Information Service, can help to fill the gap. There are also registers that list the current research in colleges and universities. The librarian will be able to help in identifying these. Some libraries run their own current awareness service.

Before you start searching the bibliographies, abstracts or indexes, one essential step is to consult the list of subject headings covered. This will be found in a separate booklet, and is important because the subject you are searching for may appear under a slightly different classification than your key word.

Another source that may prove useful are encyclopaedias. Apart from the usual *Encyclopaedia Brittanica,* there are encyclopaedias dealing with particular fields of learning, such as medicine or nursing. Again, use the skills of the librarian to help track down these and other sources of information.

COMPUTER SEARCHING

Some libraries are equipped to conduct literature searches by computer. This is a much more complex undertaking, and you will need to ask the librarian to do this for you. However, computer searches are expensive, so unless you are involved in a major piece of research it is best to try the other sources first.

Once you have obtained one or two articles or books, you will find that these contain references that you can then follow up. This is known as the 'snowball' method. In fact this can become rather dangerous and turn into more of an avalanche! It is very tempting to follow every lead in the hope it will prove useful, or because it looks interesting. Resist! Otherwise you will end up with masses of material, much of it irrelevant. Think what you are looking for, and ask yourself how the reference will contribute to the research. Once you have found a suitable reference, then the next step is to look at the original article, if the journal is taken by your library. If not, the librarian will be able to obtain a photocopy from a library in the area. If the reference is a book, then that too should be obtained. It is not sufficient just to note that certain work has been published on the subject in question, you must read the original material. When you find yourself coming across references that have already been noted, then you have probably gone far enough in that area and should move on. Literature searching can become addictive, so you need to set yourself a time limit. As a rough guide, the literature search will take between a quarter and a third of the total time available for a project.

Certain subjects may turn out to have been extensively researched already, with a considerable amount of existing literature. This does not necessarily mean that the research you plan must be abandoned, but it does mean that it will require careful thought and planning. There are two ways of coping with this situation. First, it is perfectly valid to replicate previous research. This means that the original research is repeated as closely as possible, to see if the results are repeated. Clearly, the implication of this is that the tools used, the type of sample and all other variables must match the original research. Replication is very valuable, but unfortunately does not have the glamour of original research, so is too little exercised in nursing research. The second way of dealing with this is to supply a different angle to the original work, repeating a research tool on a different sample for instance, or a different tool on the same type of sample, or testing a new theory on the same research topic. As long as you can support your new approach through logical argument and use of the literature, then there is no reason why the project should not go ahead.

Points to remember

1. Literature searching is often slow to begin with, so do not get discouraged.
2. You will need to go to more indexes if you find that there are not many references for your subject.
3. Most indexes have an author list as well as a subject list. So if you know the author of an article or book on your topic, look to see if he or she has other published work.
4. Journals have their own cumulative index, usually annually. This is useful if you know of a journal catering for a specialist need, e.g. intensive care nursing.
5. Use the reference lists at the end of books and articles.

KEEPING TRACK

Whenever you visit the library during your seach, be sure to take a notebook and pencil with you, so that you can note down references you wish to follow up. Make sure you have enough information to find the reference when you need it.

One absolutely essential thing to do is to have some system of recording the references you read. One way to do this is to use post cards or something similar as a Kardex. On one side write the title, author, date and source of publication. If this is a journal, the author, full journal title, title of the article, volume, number and page numbers must all be recorded. For books, you should record the author, title, publishing company and place of publication, e.g.

> Watson J (1981) Nursing's scientific quest. *Nursing Outlook,* **29** (7): 413–416.
> Abrams M (1977) *Beyond Three Score Years and Ten.* Mitchum: Age Concern.

On the back of the card write a brief summary of the contents, so that you can refer quickly to relevant material at a later date. Just how you catalogue is a matter of personal preference. It could be alphabetically by author, grouped by subject. You could even duplicate your references, and have one alphabetical and one by subject, then cross-reference them. If you have a computer, references can be kept on this, but make a note of just what each file on your reference disc contains or you will have to search them all each time you wish to refer to one.

Incidentally, you will find different systems for referencing in different texts. Some quote the author and date in the text, then the references are listed alphabetically and in full at the end. Others give each reference a number as it occurs in the text and they are listed in full in numerical order at the end.

Literature searching is time-consuming, frustrating and requires much patience. It is also an exciting and enriching experience.

SCENARIO

So now let's see how the ward team would tackle the literature search. It is important for them to work out who is going to do what, or they could end up all covering the same ground rather than extending and deepening the search.

As Sister Jones is interested in the possible implications of the new policy on the ward, she decides that she will look for reports on other day- and 5-day surgical schemes. This will give her some ideas about the difficulties and advantages of such policies. In addition, Sister Jones hopes to see what kind of records or other data were collected, or what other methodology was used in these studies.

The problem for Sister Brown is that her part of the project is about how patients and their relatives feel – in other words their attitudes. The librarian has already suggested that, initially, Sister Brown should seek literature on patients discharged from hospital after any illness or operation. Then it may be possible to narrow down to acute conditions.

There is so much literature nowadays on the nursing process that poor Staff Nurse Baker does not know where to start! However, she finally decides to search first for reports of situations where a change to the nursing process model of care has been carried out and monitored. She will also need to look at some of the basic texts on the philosophy behind the nursing process, and any work on how its use could be evaluated.

Student Nurse Green intends to look at the things that worry patients about going home after surgery. So she needs to search the literature for any work in which the patients' perspective was examined. There has been some work on this, but not all of it related to surgical patients. Nevertheless, Student Nurse Green will find that patients' attitudes to other types of health care may give her some ideas worth exploring in her own work. Such research may also help in her thinking on the methodology. In addition, some of the basic psychology texts might prove useful at a later stage, in considering how people cope with frightening or stressful circumstances. As this will be a qualitative study, she will need to consult research textbooks for guidance on qualitative research.

The team agree to keep a central index of references as well as their personal one, so that they can each look through the references being generated to see which are relevant to them. In addition, Sister Jones decides to ask the hospital librarian to help her compile a list of research textbooks that might be helpful.

Exercises

1. Find a piece of research written in the last 3 years on your own speciality, using the indexes, bibliographies and abstracts mentioned.
2. Find a research paper, article or book on a particular topic, but applied to your own speciality, e.g. nurse–patient communication, again using the indexes, abstracts or bibliographies.

   In a class situation, the papers can be brought to the group, with an explanation of how the individual went about searching for it, where it was actually found and any problems or false leads encountered.
3. Choose a topic in your own clinical field and conduct a literature search on this subject. How extensive you make your search will depend on the time available to you, but if this is limited then use the sources most readily accessible to you, otherwise your search could take a very long time. When you feel you have sufficient material, write up your search.

Libraries

The Royal College of Nursing Library
Extensive collection of nursing and related literature. Steinberg Collection of Theses. Information service available. Open to nurses, postal lending service to members.

The Librarian, Royal College of Nursing, 20 Cavendish Square, London W1M 0AB. Tel. 01-409 3333.

The King's Fund Library

Literature on a wide range of health-care issues. Service open to genuine enquiries.

The Librarian, King's Fund Centre, 126 Albert Street, London NW1 7NF. Tel. 01-267 6111.

The Department of Health Library

International collection on NHS, social services and social security (mostly managerial and policy). Information service open to NHS employees and genuine enquiries.

Alexander Fleming House, Elephant and Castle, London SE1 6BY. Tel. 01-407 5522.

The Scottish Health Service Centre Library

Literature on management, planning and administration of health services and related subjects. Open to all Scottish Health Service employees.

The Librarian, Scottish Health Service Centre, Crewe Rd South, Edinburgh. EH4 21F. Tel. 031-332 2335.

Bibliographies, abstracts and indexes

Royal College of Nursing Bibliography
Published monthly.

DoH Nursing Research Abstracts
Published quarterly.

DoH Health Service Abstracts
Published monthly.

American Journal of Nursing Company International Nursing Index
Published quarterly, with cumulative volume at end of year.

Index Medicus
Published quarterly. English and Foreign Language material listed on medical subjects.

BIBLIOGRAPHY

Macleod Clark J and Stodulski A (1978) How to find out: a guide to searching the literature. *Nursing Times,* **74** (6): 21–23.

Moorbath P (1988) A guide to nursing research literature. *Senior Nurse*, **8** (1): 35–36.

Pollock L (1984) 6 Steps to a successful literature search. *Nursing Times*, **80** (44): 40–43.

Treece E W and Treece J W (1986) The library and computer-based literature searches. *Elements of Research in Nursing*, ch. 7. St. Louis, Toronto, Princeton: Mosby.

4

Evaluating Published Research

SCENARIO

The team were well embarked on their literature search when Staff Nurse Baker came to the team meeting looking very gloomy.

She had read an article on the nursing process that she had found in one of the journals and had thought it very interesting and useful. Then the tutor on her diploma course had mentioned the same article and had been quite critical of several points.

The team discussed this and realised that they all had the same problem. As beginners, how could they evaluate the standard and content of the literature they were reading?

Knowing how to read research critically is one of the most useful skills a nurse can acquire, whether or not she is engaged in research. You may remember from Chapter 1 that not knowing how to evaluate research findings was one of Hunt's four reasons why nurses do not utilise research. Books and articles on research have much more meaning if read like this, so that the relevance and appropriateness of the findings to clinical practice can be better judged.

Reading and making sense of research books and articles is a bit like reading a detective story. The reader likes to be able to follow all the twists of the plot, trying to spot the clues for herself, then deciding if on the evidence collected the author was justified in coming up with the solution that he or she presents. So it is with reading research – can you follow the threads of the argument, are some things missed, and does the 'evidence' support the research conclusions?

This seems a very daunting task to the beginner. How do you know what to look for? Can you not simply take it all on trust? After all the work has been published, so it must be right, surely?

The answer is that there are almost certainly going to be elements of the work on which it is possible to hold different views. Besides, it is you the reader who needs to be convinced about the strength of the case. You want to know whether the research reported is valid and reliable. Only then will you be able to judge its relevance and application for yourself.

The main thing to bear in mind is that the author has (or should have) gone through the research process in carrying out the work reported on. So by thinking about how the author went through the various stages, there is a framework for the investigations. The key questions you need to ask are:

1. What was the study about?
2. Why was it done?
3. How was it done?
4. Are the findings explained, justified and relevant?

WHAT WAS THE STUDY ABOUT?

One of the difficulties in reviewing literature is that it is not always possible to decide what a work is all about by the title. How descriptive is the title of the work, then? An abstract or summary can help to show quickly whether or not it is relevant for your needs by giving an impression of the contents, so is there an abstract? Was the research worthwhile – is it a subject that is of concern and interest to nurses and nursing, or to other health-care disciplines?

WHY WAS THE STUDY DONE?

Does the paper explain why the writer chose to study that particular question? It could have been that it arose from his or her work, but does it say so? How the writer became involved in the subject in the first place can tell you how experienced he or she was, both in the field under study and in conducting research. This latter point is important, as the research could have been conducted by someone very inexperienced in research techniques. This clearly will affect the quality of the work. Should this seem to be the case, then is there any explanation of how the researcher was supervised – was there a supervisor or supervisory board? If the research was sponsored or funded by a particular body, it could have had an influence on the research, so it is relevant to know how the research was funded. Just why was the research question formulated in the first place, and is the problem, research objective or hypothesis clearly stated? Was there a Steering Committee who might have been influential in such decisions?

HOW WAS IT DONE?

First of all, what kind of research design was it, survey, interpretative or experimental? The design should always be appropriate to the research question, so ask yourself whether you feel this is so.

Another area to examine is the literature review. Look at the dates of the references – are they very old or are there some recent references also? If the topic is well known to you, you will be able to judge whether the review has included the most recent and important work or whether there are some serious omissions. How do the references and literature appear to have been used: do they add to the arguments being presented or have they been 'tacked on' to give an appearance of scholarship to the work?

The author should also have clearly defined the terms used: how was 'non-compliance with diet' or other variables interpreted for the purpose of the research? Is that definition sensible?

If the research involved the use of a sample of any kind, the work should discuss how it was chosen, whether it was representative of the study population and whether it was adequate in size for the purpose.

The reasons for the rejection of possible alternative methods should be discussed, together with the pros and cons of the method that were used. Any research tools such as questionnaires should be explained as far as their origin and testing are concerned, and if a pilot study was conducted, whether changes were subsequently made. A full report should contain copies of measurement tools, usually as an appendix, but in an article one or two 'specimen' questions or part of the attitude scale gives some flavour of the actual data collection method.

One of the areas sometimes unexplored in research publications is the ethical considerations of the study. It is worth thinking about ethical issues that you feel could have been involved. Does the author discuss these and is there evidence of respondents being given the choice as to whether or not to participate?

ARE THE RESULTS EXPLAINED, JUSTIFIED AND RELEVANT?

For a start, the paper should contain an explanation of just how the data were analysed. This applies to both qualitative and quantitative data. The use of computers in the analysis should be acknowledged and information given as to the nature of statistical advice or supervision as appropriate.

When it comes to the results themselves, the thing to ask yourself is can you as the reader understand them? Are tables and graphs clearly labelled and can you work out what they are telling you? Do not be blinded by science – if you cannot make sense of the information presented then the author has failed in his or her basic task – communication and enlightenment.

Sometimes, one or two statistical tests are given. Obviously, you will not be able to interpret these without some statistical knowledge. Chapter 11 will examine quantitative data, and explain some of the statistical techniques used in its analysis. It is worth making yourself acquainted with the more frequently used tests, then you can form your own impression as to the validity of the results. Even the use of percentages is worth examination.

For example, if raw numbers are not given as well, the reader may not be made aware that the impressive figure of 90% for instance actually refers to 9 people, where the total sample was 10.

Having examined the data, do you feel that the author is justified in drawing the conclusions given? Go back to the stated hypothesis or research objectives to see how the results relate to these. There may well be gaps, omissions or assumptions, but, if so, these should be acknowledged and discussed. Look out for quantum leaps between the data and the conclusions drawn from them!

Finally, if the work included recommendations, either for research or for policy, do you consider that they are supported by the research? Do they flow from the findings or appear to have been put in as an afterthought? Above all, are you convinced enough to implement them?

SUMMARY

The aim of reading research in this way is not to tear it to pieces and discard it, as there is always something to learn from any study. The aim is to make a reasoned judgment about the research. This takes skill and practice, but the questions to ask can be put into a check-list:

1. *Research problem.* Is this stated in clear terms, and the reason for its generation explained?
2. *Influences, assumptions and limitations.* Could the funding organisation, the nature of the research or the background and experience of the researcher have biased the results? Who gave advice or supervised the project?
3. *Literature and references.* How up to date and comprehensive is the researcher's knowledge of the subject? Is the literature well integrated into the arguments presented? Are theoretical concepts, if any, adequately discussed?
4. *Research objectives and hypothesis.* How well do they relate to the original research problem?
5. *Description of study.* Is it clear whether the study is experimental, survey or interpretative? Is the nature of the population, the size of the sample and the definition of variables given?
6. *Research methodology.* Why was that particular method chosen? How were research tools developed and are there examples of them? What was the response rate?
7. *Pilot study.* Were changes made on the basis of the pilot study? If there was no pilot study, why was this?
8. *Ethical issues.* What ethical issues are relevant to the study, and how were these taken into account?
9. *Data analysis.* What form did this take? What statistical tests have been conducted? Can the reader understand the results fairly easily?

10. *Conclusions and recommendations.* How do these relate to the research aims? If all research aims have not been met, is this discussed? Has the hypothesis been proven? Could alternative hypotheses provide a better explanation of the results? Are the recommendations justified by the research as presented?

RESEARCH TERMINOLOGY

One of the stumbling blocks to reading research or writing up your own is that there are certain ways of expressing things that to the lay person sound like jargon. This is not surprising as research, like any other tradition of scholarship, has developed its own language, the purpose of which is not to mystify the reader but to enable practitioners to communicate more easily. Unfortunately, the existence of this research language means that it is all too easy for research publications to be written in a style that is unintelligible to many readers, creating an elitist perception of research and a gap between the researcher and the nurse practitioner that does the cause of true nursing research no good at all. The best defence against this is to become familiar with research terminology and its usage. A glossary of research terms is given at the end of the book.

RESEARCH AWARENESS

Once you have learned how to read research critically, you will find that it alters your whole attitude to the nursing literature. The relevance and possible application to your speciality of the articles and books that you read becomes much more apparent and the findings and conclusions make far more sense. At this point, you may find yourself beginning to collect copies of articles that interest you. The danger is that you will slowly sink under a mountain of paper unless you find a way of organising yourself and the material you read.

The easiest way to do this is to start a research awareness file. As the name implies, it is a file that is designed to keep you abreast of current developments in your field. One method of doing this is to get into the habit of looking through some of the bibliographies and indexes discussed in Chapter 3 at intervals, maybe every 3 months or so. Or you could arrange with colleagues that each of you will scan a certain journal regularly and then pool your findings as the staff on ward 4 decide to do. Having listed the references that seem interesting, gradually read them in turn, and with your newly acquired critical facilities pick out the ones that you feel have most to offer. Then catalogue them as described, with a brief account of the contents on the back. You may decide to start a research awareness board on the ward on which interesting references or photocopies of articles are pinned for everyone to see. You could either destroy the references to the articles you reject or keep them separately in case you have a need for them at a later date. In practice, it is probably safer to take the latter course because if you destroy references it is almost a certainty that you will need them one day!

SCENARIO

The ward team decide to try a critique of an article together so that they will be in a better position when it comes to understanding the literature they are reading. The paper they choose is given below. You might like to try it yourself, before seeing what the ward team thought.

RESEARCH CRITIQUE EXAMPLAR OF 'WHERE ARE THEY NOW? A SURVEY OF CAREER PATTERNS OF DIPLOMA IN NURSING HOLDERS' by Brenda Bedford RGN DPSN

Background

The Diploma in Nursing Studies requires a working understanding and appreciation of research and its application and implications for nursing practice. In order to gain a greater understanding of research principles, the students on the diploma course at Hightown College of Further Education were required to conduct a research-based project during the final two terms of the course.

Discussions took place in class with the tutors who were to supervise the projects concerning the research topics that students wished to explore. During one of these sessions the question came up of the extent to which the diploma course changed the career plans of those completing the course. The author decided to make this the topic of her project.

The research was planned around two main assumptions:

1. Gaining a nursing diploma (DPSN or the London Diploma in Nursing) would stimulate nurses to make changes in their professional lives, either by moving away from the bedside and into nurse education, management or research or by taking further studies.
2. There would be more changes in the career patterns of men than of women.

The review of the literature was conducted using the nursing indexes and bibliographies, and an on-line computer search was conducted with the help of the librarian to find additional references.

Several recent studies had traced the career paths of students from post-basic nursing courses. Rogers[1] found that a high proportion of JBCNS Certificate holders wished to stay in a clinical post. Montague and Herbert[2] and Kemp[3] showed a tendency for nursing degree graduates to stay in clinical nursing for the first few years. A commitment to continuing higher education and research activity was also shown by the graduates and in studies of nursing education and nursing administration students by Hardy et al[4] and Sinclair et al[5]. Hardy noted that male students outnumbered female students on the nursing education certificate course.

Method

With the assumptions of the project and the literature in mind, a questionnaire was drafted which was 'piloted' on diploma holders locally and checked with statistical staff at the college. The final draft of the questionnaire included closed and open questions so that questions could be analysed both quantitatively and qualitatively.

A sample of 20 diploma courses was selected by stratified random sampling to cover proportional numbers of DPSN and London diploma courses at colleges and schools of nursing throughout the UK. To preserve confidentiality, each course was sent 10 questionnaires, with envelopes, and asked to distribute them to a range of diploma students from the last 10 years (total of 200 questionnaires). The response to the survey was over 65%, even though no follow-up letter was possible.

Returned questionnaires were coded with the aid of a computer studies student, who also participated in the data analysis by SPSSX at a computer terminal, guided by the computer staff at the college.

Results

The results will be discussed with reference to the two main assumptions:

Assumption 1

It had been assumed that gaining the diploma would stimulate nurses to make changes in their professional lives, either by moving away from the bedside and into education, management or research, or by undertaking further studies. Of all respondents, 65% had had a change in career since the diploma and 46% felt this change had been influenced by the course.

Figure 4.1 shows career patterns of diploma holders before, during and after gaining the diploma. There is a significant shift away from the clinical area to education and management, particularly education. (The category 'other' includes full-time courses, non-health care, family or missing data.)

When respondents were asked about their future career the trend continued: 18% anticipated that they would be in clinical work (including community nursing), with 40% aiming for education jobs and 12% for management, 15% were in the 'other' category and another 15% were 'don't knows'.

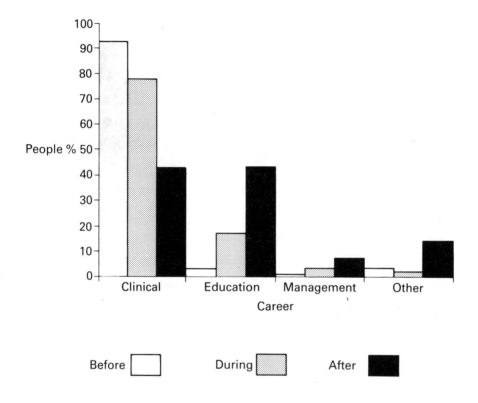

Figure 4.1   Careers before, during and after the diploma

Comments on the questionnaire relating to career moves were analysed qualitatively and provided some explanations for the quantitative results. Many respondents had taken the diploma course because they wanted to enter nurse education, using the course either for direct entry to a nurse tutor course or just as a prerequisite or 'stepping stone' towards a teaching qualification. Sometimes the course was offered in conjunction with clinical teacher training.

Many others said that although they had started the diploma to improve or update their clinical practice, the course had decided them to go into teaching. So the diploma did prove to be a turning point in careers away from clinical and management posts. For example:

The Diploma pushed me away from management to education.

One respondent said she looked towards education because of:

A need for individual responsibility not fulfilled in clinical nursing.

Others commented:

The Diploma increased awareness of education skills needed to promote changes in practice.

Became aware of need for changes in attitudes which led to teaching career.

With regard to diploma holders becoming involved in further studies, research, etc., 63% of the sample had progressed to higher education (first and second degrees, other diploma courses, education certificates), 33% had engaged in research and 16% had had work published. Examples of the value of the diploma as a preparation for further study were cited in the comments. One student gained the confidence to apply for a health visitor course 'even though my age was against me'. Another took a psychology degree because she had enjoyed the subject so much on the diploma course. Several respondents commented on their ambition to proceed to a nursing degree.

Assumption 2

The extent to which men would show more changes in career patterns than women was also examined. In fact only 18% of men changed jobs compared to 61% of women, but as Figure 4.2 shows there is a more marked shift among men towards education and management after the diploma course. Twice as many women as men stay in clinical nursing and these number more than the women in the two other main areas. On the other hand, there are more men than women in education than in the other areas.

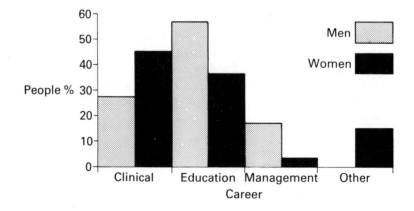

Figure 4.2   Careers after the diploma for men and women

Again the trend continues when respondents were asked about their future career. In 5 years' time only 4% of men intended to be in clinical nursing, compared to 23% of women. Of those currently engaged in further education courses, 35% were women and 59% were men.

All the differences between men and women respondents were statistically significant.

Characteristics of the sample

The ratio of women to men in the sample was 77:23. The median age of respondents was 35. Seventy-five per cent of the sample were RGN/SRN qualified and 20% RMN (5% 'missing' or 'other'), the median year of basic qualification being 1977. Sixty-two per cent had at least one post-basic qualification and 10% had four. Nearly all were full-time employees.

Discussion

The results of this project were tending to confirm the two original assumptions. There were trends in the career patterns of the diploma students and these were stronger among the male respondents in the sample. Yet some of the findings contradicted those from the literature. The study showed a drift away from clinical practice after diploma training, whereas other similar research (Rogers, Montague and Herbert, Kemp) suggested that students remain clinicians. The explanation might be found in a comparison of age and experience. The nursing diploma courses are post-basic so, therefore, applicants tend to be mature, already have some years of experience and may be at a point of change. The sample indeed showed a mature range of ages from 27 to 56, with a variety of backgrounds, compared with the usual age of nursing graduates at the beginning of their career. The comments made by respondents also lend support to this conclusion.

The findings on sex differences certainly support those of Hardy who found that male students outnumber females on nursing education courses. There are also parallels between these findings and Hardy's in terms of the number of students who go on to research activity.

References

1. Rogers J (1983) The impact of post-basic clinical education. *Nursing Times,* **79** (17): 42–44.
2. Montague S E and Herbert R A (1982) Career paths of graduates of a degree-linked nursing course. *Journal of Advanced Nursing*, **7**: 359–370.
3. Kemp J (1985) The graduate's progress. *Nursing Times,* **81** (49): 42–43.
4. Hardy L K, Sinclair H and Hughes J (1984) Nursing careers: findings of a follow-up survey of graduates of the nursing education and administration certificate

courses of the Department of Nursing Studies, University of Edinburgh, 1958-1975. *Journal of Advanced Nursing,* **9**: 611–618.
5. Sinclair H C, Hardy L K and Hughes J (1984) Educational achievement of nurses who completed the nursing education and the nursing administration certificate courses of the Department of Nursing Studies, University of Edinburgh, 1958-1975. *Journal of Advanced Nursing,* **9**: 603–609.

CRITIQUE OF STUDY

What is your view of this paper? One thing to bear in mind is that the purpose of a critique is not to demolish the research, but to look for both the good and the not-so-good points and to think how the findings – whatever they were or however limited – could be used or built upon.

Purpose of the research

Bedford makes it quite clear that this research was undertaken primarily as a student assignment, to provide a learning experience for a particular group of students. As such, rigour in the execution of the research could potentially have been at risk through lack of experience. Whereas this problem appears to have been overcome in the actual conduct of the research, the limitations of student projects are apparent in some areas.

Development of research design and use of the literature

The initiation and development of the research is well explained, and supervision by a course tutor has clearly resulted in a carefully executed project. What is somewhat unusual is the way in which two assumptions are used as the basis for the research. More could have been made of the contradictions that were identified in the existing literature and which could have led to the construction of a number of reasoned hypotheses. This feature is particularly surprising given the use of a questionnaire as the research tool and the intention to employ statistical techniques for analysis. Such a research design lends itself admirably to hypothesis testing and would have made more direct use of the statistical results.

Methodology

The sampling frame and sample were well constructed and justified by the research aims. As this was a postal questionnaire, the use of closed questions was sensible, whereas the inclusion of open questions provided respondents with the opportunity to express an opinion more fully.

What is lacking in the explanation of the method is why a control group was not used. What reasons were there for assuming that the career pattern of diploma students was different from that of their contemporaries who did not take the diploma course? This seems a serious omission if the purpose of the research was to examine changes brought about by exposure to the experiences of the diploma course and this does seem to be the case.

Presentation of results

The results presented are somewhat sparse, given that a tool as powerful as SPSSX was used for the analysis. The labelling of Figure 4.1 does not make it entirely clear that each set of bars relates to the careers from which students on the diploma course came. This being so, the changes in careers that do indeed appear to have occurred could have been more clearly illustrated. The data presented concerning differences between men and women suffers from having no comparison with a control group. There is some evidence that male nurses as a group do aim their careers towards education and management.

Discussion

The explanation for the contradictions between the research findings and that of previous work is the greater degree of maturity of students undertaking the diploma course. What has not been clearly demonstrated is that the changes in career that were identified in diploma students were significantly different from those of nurses of similar maturity but who did not take the diploma course.

Summary

The project presented was no doubt an invaluable learning exercise. The research was competently executed and resulted in some interesting find-ings. What was it about the diploma course that brought about the change in career, for example, and did the course attract students who were already looking for further stimulation in their working environment? However, the limitations of the research design mean that it lacks reliability. The findings do, however, provide several potentially fruitful avenues for further research.

Exercises

1. Choose a short paper and prepare a short critique on it, as if you were presenting it to a group of colleagues. Imagine that the presentation is to last no more than 10 minutes.
2. Choose a research-based paper and write a critique of approximately 1000 words. If possible, it is best if the paper chosen is on an area of

nursing with which you are familiar, as then you can approach the work with some degree of knowledge of the subject.

These two exercises are set at different levels of difficulty, so that you can become familiar with the techniques in the first exercise, then proceed to a more structured approach. In a group setting the short critique could be conducted by individuals and then presented and discussed in class, or two or three people could work together in preparing a critique for presentation and discussion with others.

BIBLIOGRAPHY

Abdellah F and Levine C (1979) Analysis and interpretation of research findings. *Better Patient Care Through Nursing Research,* pp. 409–413. New York: Macmillan.

Chapman C C (1984) Evaluating published research. *The Research Process in Nursing,* ed. D F S Cormack, ch. 20. Oxford: Blackwell Scientific Publications.

Fox D J (1976) Critically evaluating the written research report. *Fundamentals of Research in Nursing,* ch. 13. New York: Appleton-Century-Crofts.

Hawthorn P J (1983) Principles of research: a checklist. *Nursing Times,* Occasional Paper, **79** (35): 41–43.

Hunt J (1984) Research: step by step. *Nursing Mirror,* **158** (1): 29–30.

Notter L (1979) The evaluation process. *Essentials of Research in Nursing,* ch. 11. London: Tavistock Publications.

Treece E W and Treece J W (1986) Critiquing an article and critiquing skills. *Research in Nursing,* ch. 4. St Louis, Toronto, Princeton: Mosby.

Walker J (1984) Making sense of investigation. *Nursing Mirror,* **158** (10): 15–16.

5

Research Design

Research needs to be carefully planned if it is to have any credibility and usefulness. A research proposal is usually prepared to act as a means of informing others about just what is intended and to help channel the researcher's own thoughts. It acts as a 'blueprint' for the research. Writing a research proposal is quite an exacting task and should be tackled in a systematic way: Chapter 12 explains how to do this in detail. The first step, however, is to consider the overall plan of the study and how it will be carried out. This plan is known as the research design. So our ward team need to spend some time thinking about their research design before they go any further. Needless to say, they all have different thoughts about just what the design should be.

SCENARIO

The ward team hold a meeting to decide how they will go about the research they plan to conduct. The question that causes the most difficulty is what methods to use.

Sister Jones has always been more interested in the scientific component of nursing. She likes to feel that her decisions are based on rational arguments and carefully proven facts. So her immediate ideas are to concentrate on collecting very specific information that will, she assumes, speak for itself. Besides, Sister considers that her managers will only be convinced by facts and figures. However, although personal inclination and talents are bound to play a part in research design, they are by no means the overriding factors.

The community nurse, Sister Brown, is not so sure which kind of methods to use. She agrees with Sister Jones that sound reasoning and clear evidence are necessary but feels that people are too complex and their actions too complicated to reduce to a set of numbers and display of tables. How will patients feel about the new policy? If patients or their relatives are not able to cope with earlier discharge, that will have an effect on her work.

Staff Nurse Baker agrees with Sister about the need to be scientific but wonders whether some kind of experiment is possible. After all, the whole point of experiments is to prove things surely?

Student Nurse Green has heard a little about qualitative research. In fact, she has to carry out a small research project using qualitative methods as an assignment for the research methods course her nurse training school has just introduced for third-year students. What she is not sure about is just which method to use and how reliable the information will be.

CHOOSING METHODS

Discussions about what kind of research to carry out and which methods are more reliable become quite heated at times! So how is the dilemma to be resolved? The team are forgetting that the decision about the approach to use must be made taking into account the purpose of the research and what would be the most appropriate to achieve that.

Since the earliest development of research in nursing there has been debate about the nature of such research. Early nurse researchers had no traditions or examples on which to build, so understandably turned to the natural sciences as a model. Also, if the new discipline was to be taken seriously then it had to be seen to be 'scientific' and 'respectable'.

One of the criticisms that used to be made of nursing research was that nursing had no theory-base of its own so had to 'borrow' from other disciplines, such as education, sociology or psychology. Why does this matter – isn't it enough just to gather the information required in order to answer the research question?

The answer is that it is not that straightforward. As any nurse would point out, nursing is not just a science. Carper (1978) identified 4 types of nursing knowledge:

1. Empirics – the science of nursing.
2. Aesthetics – the art of nursing.
3. Personal knowledge.
4. Ethics or moral knowledge.

Hockey (1986) described nursing as 'the art of applying nursing knowledge'. Nurses have been trying to define just what nursing is since Florence Nightingale's day and will no doubt continue to do so. Clearly both art and science have to be taken into account, but what nurses do at any one time is likely to be somewhere along a continuum ranging from pure art to pure science.

Art _____ Science

Research studies will vary also according to whether they are orientated towards theory or practice.

Theory _____ Practice

Where one is along these lines in nursing research will depend on the purpose of the research, the experience, knowledge and clinical speciality of the person concerned.

At one end of the continuum you have the studies that are purely about increasing knowledge. Examples of this would be studies of nurse–patient communication (Wells, 1980). At the other end of the continuum are the studies concerned mainly with suggesting and implementing changes in practice (Rodin, 1983). Of course, theoretical research is intended to influence practice and practical research is based on theory. There is also research that combines both approaches. The various nursing models are examples of this. They generate nursing theory while providing a guide to practice. You may also come across the terms 'basic' and 'applied', which are used to describe the two main approaches.

Weiss (1977) has talked about the nature of research, both theoretical and practical, that attempts to influence policy. He distinguishes between decision-driven and knowledge-driven models of policy research. Decision-driven research is often commissioned to help in decision-making. Knowledge-driven research is more theoretical, but has often been found to have more influence on policy change in the long term than the decision-driven approach.

This seems to suggest that nurse researchers should beware of becoming 'hired hacks'. There is a danger that the researcher is forced to accept the policy-makers' definition of the problem and to provide the answers they require. Research should involve a degree of academic freedom. The nurse researcher needs to keep in touch with theoretical bases and be continually challenging and negotiating. Nursing as a discipline draws knowledge from a wide range of sources each with its own style of research. The potential choice of research styles or methods for nursing research is, therefore, very wide and ranges from the highly quantitative methods of the biological and medical sciences, through the social sciences and humanities to more qualitative methods, and relates also to the art–science continuum referred to earlier.

Quantitative ——————————————————— Qualitative
methods   methods

Biological and
medical sciences ———— Social sciences ———— Humanities

Quantitative research is concerned primarily with measurement of facts – about people, events or things – and establishing the strength of the relationship between variables, usually by statistics (the number-crunching approach), so data are in the form of numbers. Large-scale research on large groups of people, all nurses who qualified in a certain year and their subsequent career patterns for example, would use quantitative methods to collect large amounts of data, but small research projects may also be best conducted in this way. The theory behind quantitative research is that only by employing such methods can confidence be placed on the results and the hypothesis be adequately tested. Quantitative research is sometimes described as providing hard data.

Qualitative research is based on the rationale that human behaviour can only be understood by getting to know the perspective and interpretation of events of the person or people being studied – by seeing things through their eyes – rather than by reliance on the measurement of concrete facts. So the data here are mainly in word rather than number form. In this it follows the tradition of anthropologists and sociologists. Qualitative methods may be used for a complete study or may be used before a quantitative study (e.g. a survey) or after a quantitative study (to explain a statistical relationship).

FIT OF THEORY AND METHOD

Whichever type of research design is decided upon, and no matter just where along the research spectrum a project is, it will be strengthened and enhanced if it is related to an appropriate theoretical framework. The theoretical basis of research guides the formulation of an appropriate hypothesis, indicates the type of data required and hence the methodology most suitable to the topic and provides a means of understanding and interpreting the data collected. Whereas research that is not related to theory may provide interesting information, but cannot contribute to the wider body of knowledge. The explanation that you feel fits your data is limited to that study and those data alone. It is not generalisable.

Theories are developed from systematic formal research, which provides an increasing body of knowledge about the complex relationships between people and their environment.

Theory is classified as *inductive* or *deductive*.

Inductive theory is not concerned with testing out presumed associations or saying what is likely to happen. Inductive research starts with specific observations or events, moves to more generalised ideas regarding concepts and possible relationships and thence to generating theory.

Deductive theory works the other way round – starting with a particular theory and inferring the probable relationships between variables in a given situation.

Inductive theory
particular case (observed data) ⟶ testable hypothesis ⟶ generalised theory

Deductive theory
generalised theory ⟶ testable hypothesis ⟶ particular case

Although inductive and deductive theory have been described as though they were two distinct phenomena, this is far from the case. Inductive reasoning may be used to explain why certain things occurred – if some diabetic patients stick to their diet and some do not, a theory about 'self' from psychology may perhaps explain the differences.

The theory may be then used deductively to suggest how other patients may behave – amputees' determination to regain mobility, for example.

Theories then can describe, explain, predict or prescribe.

Theory used to describe

If you remember from the 'getting started' chapter, one of the questions posed was 'what is going on here?'. Much research is descriptive in that it seeks to answer that type of question. Once the research has been conducted, a particular theory may help to interpret the findings, by describing in a structured way just what is happening. For example, in her study of nurse–patient communication in surgical wards, Macleod Clark (1983) considered that the limited nature of the conversations that were analysed could best be understood in relation to nurses' tendency to distance themselves from patients.

Theory used to explain

Although describing a situation may be sufficient in some contexts, often there is a need to look for the reason behind the situation. Theory can provide an explanation; for instance, Bond (1983) used theories related to non-disclosure of their condition to patients suffering from cancer to explain the way nurses 'managed' the nurse–patient interaction.

Theory used to predict

If theories can provide an explanation of why things happen, then theories can also predict what will happen, given a specific set of circumstances. Some research sets out to test whether such a prediction holds good. Webb (1983), in an experimental design, predicted from existing theory concerning coping mechanisms that women given an information and support counselling session following hysterectomy would recover more quickly and be more satisfied with their care.

Theory used to prescribe

As we have said before in this book, one of the criticisms of nursing research and of nursing in general is that it has no true theory of its own. If you think back to earlier chapters, one of the reasons for getting involved in research is to provide reasoned and rational explanations for the care we give to patients. Theory can be used to decide just what nursing care will be the most effective. For instance, educational theory may be employed by the nurse to decide what form a teaching programme for renal patients being dialysed should take if it is to succeed. Theories concerning stress and coronary heart disease can guide the nurse in the information she gives to patients attending a well-person clinic. Utilising research findings in this way is perhaps the challenge facing nursing at present.

How does this affect research design? The point is that at the design stage, in fact even before that, the question to be answered is do you develop or utilise a theory and then collect data that seek to support it or do you collect data first then try to develop a theory to fit or adapt an existing theory? Clearly, if you are trying to test theory that seems relevant to your particular subject of interest, you will set out to collect the kind of data that will verify or refute that theory (prediction). On the other hand, if you collect the data first, the limitations of the data and the kind of data you collect will itself to some extent dictate the range of theory that will fit your particular data (description or explanation). Theory may guide the method but the method will limit or control the resulting theory.

As in many things in research, there is no clear-cut answer. Theory both precedes and follows research. It precedes by guiding the thinking on the factors that are important to investigate in research. It follows because it helps to set the research in the context of other research. So it both indicates the research direction and determines how isolated findings relate to the more abstract body of knowledge.

Research then can both originate from and contribute to theory.

Glaser and Strauss (1967) have written extensively on grounded theory, which is theory derived from and verified by the data in a continuous process. As explanatory theory begins to emerge, data are collected which will support, refute or refine this theory. This is arguably more credible than explaining data arising from one research enterprise by theory originating from another. Grounded theory is explained more fully in Chapter 8.

Nurses are beginning to develop theories of nursing, but must not fall into the trap of taking these theories as sacrosanct. As a mature discipline, nursing must have the confidence to put theory to the test.

The continuum between quantitative and qualitative methods can be represented by the three main research styles that are available to the researcher:

Quantitative _____ Qualitative

Experiment _____ Survey _____ Interpretative

Each of these is described briefly with some examples and comments on their advantages and disadvantages.

EXPERIMENTAL METHODS

Measurements are made under conditions of systematic control of different features (variables) of a research setting.

Not all experiments are carried out by white-coated men in laboratories. There are different kinds of experimental designs, but the simplest way of thinking about it is the classic 'before and after' model. A sample of patients is chosen and measurements on some variables are taken – knowledge of their special diet requirements for example. Then some manipulation takes place – a teaching programme, say – then the measurement is repeated. The aim of the experiment would be to see whether the patients' knowledge of diet is improved by planned teaching. Experimental design is discussed in Chapter 6.

Pros: Allows strong conclusions to be drawn about the cause and effect of the variables under study.
Cons: Social settings do not usually permit the application of experiments. Thus they are often conducted in 'artificial' situations. There are also ethical issues in conducting research on people, no matter how harmless the procedures to be employed appear.

SURVEY METHODS

These use questionnaires, tests and interviews with large samples of the population. This is sometimes called descriptive research because it describes what is going on. Birch (1975) used survey in studying the career patterns of student nurses.

Pros: Information can be collected quickly and comparatively cheaply.
Cons: The information may be superficial.

INTERPRETATIVE METHODS

These use observations and interviews in natural settings. Towell's work (1975) on psychiatric nursing is a classic example of this.

Pros: Produces in-depth data on the interpretations of the research setting by participants.
Cons: Time consuming. Over-identification by researcher with research setting. Findings may not apply to other settings.

Obviously these are only very broad definitions. Variations and combinations of the styles exist along the continuum. In addition, there are some other methods that do not neatly fit these categories. Although it is unlikely that you would want to use them when you are starting out in research, it is useful to know a little about such methods in case you come across examples when you are reading research papers. For convenience sake we have called these alternative methods.

ALTERNATIVE METHODS

Historical research

Medical and nursing knowledge is constantly developing at an increasing rate. At first glance then it would seem that historical research is a waste of time, but this is definitely not so. For some research questions it is impossible to study what is happening now and what may happen in the future without looking at what has happened in the past. Understanding the reasons behind the present situation can provide vital clues about the effect of and attitudes to future plans and policies. This is particularly true of more 'social' issues, such as attitudes to the mentally ill or mentally handicapped. How do you conduct research into the past? Some of the methods below are useful.

Case and life histories

For example, case or life histories, which we will examine in Chapter 8, can be historical. Asking people to relate things that happened to them during certain periods of their life can help to build up a picture of the conditions that existed at that time. By examining a number of such histories, it is possible to come to more comprehensive conclusions about the social policies that were in operation, what led to them and the consequences of these policies. This technique gives very rich data, which come 'straight from the horse's mouth' so to speak, but you have no doubt realised that the biggest problem with this type of data is the accuracy of the respondents' recall if the account is retrospective. This is less of a problem if the research is conducted as the events occur, but it still places a lot of reliance on the version of events given by those relating their 'history'.

Use of documents

It may be possible to check the information you obtain in this way by the use of documents. There are a variety of documents that can be utilised in research, whether it is historical or not. At a personal level, letters, diaries and engagement and address books can all provide data, either to verify a verbal account or on their own. Public documents include newspapers, magazines, committee minutes, reports, official statements and press releases. It is better to trace the original source of such documents if possible. A first-hand account of an event is more accurate than hearsay.

Content analysis

This method is really a particular way of using documents, or rather, two ways:
1. Counting the number of times a particular variable is mentioned in certain documents. The times the shortage of nursing staff is mentioned in national newspapers is a good example.

2.   The content or manner in which a variable is treated in particular documents. Are nurses always portrayed as 'ministering angels' for instance, and has this changed over time? Or do some newspapers do this but not others?

All the types of document listed above can be the subject of content analysis. Just which you choose will depend on the purpose of your research. The data gathered can be analysed quantitatively if they are of the first type or qualitatively if of the second. Following chapters will tell you more about analysis of quantitative and qualitative data.

Critical incidents

There are three kinds of critical incident material:

1.   Such things as accident or incident reports or patient or staff complaints. If a particular ward was reporting an increased number of patient accidents or was the subject of several complaints from ex-patients, it is an indication that all is not well on that ward. By examining this type of information, perhaps comparing one ward with another, trends over time or the precipitating cause, the researcher may be able to draw some conclusions about the clinical area under study.

2.   Another critical incident technique is to ask people to rank a list of incidents in order of importance. Is making the beds more important to a nurse than comforting a distressed patient? By applying the list to a number of respondents the researcher hopes to gain some idea of the value system and attitudes in the area under study.

3.   By asking people to describe certain events that were particularly successful (or unsuccessful), it is possible to analyse just what it was about the way the event occurred that made it a success. For example, asking sets of students to describe what a lecturer did in a lecture that they considered particularly good would enable the researcher to identify things lecturers should do to make other lectures successful – breaking the material down into small steps, encouraging the class to ask questions, for instance. This is known as Flanagan's Critical Incident Technique.

Delphi system

The Ancient Greeks used to go to Delphi to consult the oracle. Fortunately the Delphi technique does not require you to do this! But it is about consulting experts.

The way this is done is that a panel of experts are asked (by post) to give their opinion on a particular issue, perhaps by ranking items in order of importance or some kind of attitude scaling. The results are analysed and returned to all those participating (though in a non-attributable manner). Then they are asked to complete a new instrument, developed from the findings of the first round. The second time they will, of course, know how others on the panel responded so they may modify their answers in the light of this. This analysis and repeat response may be repeated up to four times. The aim is to arrive at a concensus of 'expert' opinion.

The advantage of this method is that you can gain the views of experts whom it would be difficult to interview individually. The disadvantage is that it can be costly (stationery and postage), and how up to date are the experts anyway?

Game simulation

The intention behind game simulation is that in setting up some form of game – perhaps a type of role play – people will respond in the same way as they would in real life. It is difficult to prove to what extent this is true and such games need very careful handling on the part of the researcher if they are not to cause great distress or anxiety to the participants. If you have ever taken part in this sort of exercise on a course, you will no doubt recognise this problem from your own experience, but on the other hand it may be the only way in which access to certain situations can be obtained.

Computer modelling

This very sophisticated method requires considerable computer skill to conduct. The researcher sets up a particular set of variables interacting in a certain relationship. Then one or other of the variables is changed and its effect on the others measured. The management consultants who advised the UKCC on Project 2000 used this technique to see what would be the effect on the numbers of nurses if certain situations existed, a change of entry qualification for example or a different percentage of non-practising qualified nurses returning to the NHS.

The advantage of this method is that it enables the researcher to set up situations and test out relationships and hypotheses in a way that would be impossible or difficult in real life. The disadvantage, as with any computer usage, is that if you put rubbish in you get rubbish out!

One-way mirrors

There are very obvious ethical problems with this method, so the benefits expected to result from such a project should be clear and unambiguous. One-way mirrors are sometimes used in assessing a child's reaction to various stimuli, or how the child interacts with toys or with others. As with game simulation, it may be the only way in which to get near to the actual behaviour or attitudes.

So it is not a question of 'which method should I use?' but rather one of 'which research approach is most suitable for my research question?', and then 'what research technique is most likely to give me the data (information) that I need?' (Figure 5.1).

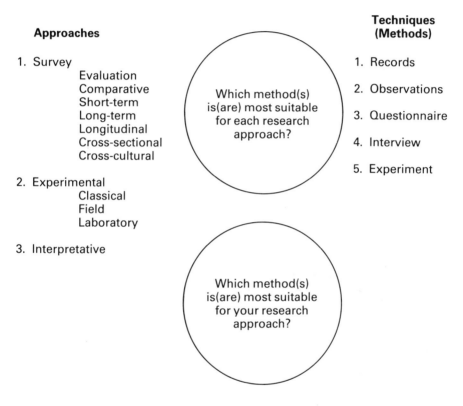

Approaches

1. Survey
    Evaluation
    Comparative
    Short-term
    Long-term
    Longitudinal
    Cross-sectional
    Cross-cultural

2. Experimental
    Classical
    Field
    Laboratory

3. Interpretative

Techniques (Methods)

1. Records

2. Observations

3. Questionnaire

4. Interview

5. Experiment

Which method(s) is(are) most suitable for each research approach?

Which method(s) is(are) most suitable for your research approach?

Figure 5.1 Approach–method relationships in research

The actual research methods listed in Figure 5.1 will be expanded in later chapters, but you can see from the figure how the method must flow from the approach that is appropriate to the research question, rather than be an isolated decision based on personal preference and narrow thinking.

The question of whether to use qualitative or quantitative methods will be largely resolved by thinking first about the research approach and techniques that are most appropriate. If the research is of an exploratory nature, trying to find out what is going on in a given situation, quantitative techniques such as a structured questionnaire would not be appropriate.

There may be very little literature on the subject, so theories that will form the framework may not be valid or contain unsubstantiated assumptions.

Quantitative research looks to existing theory in deducing the likely explanation in the relationship between variables that the research sets out to establish. The experimental model described by Webb (1983) is a quantitative method in which the relationship between the teaching programme and the increase in patient knowledge is being tested.

Qualitative research, by focusing on the respondents' perspectives, formulates theories, explanations and hypotheses during and after data collection by induction. The theory thus evolved is relevant to the specific time and setting of the research study. Research that aims to find out about attitudes – how nurses feel about caring for the dying for example – requires qualitative methods, perhaps interviews.

Whichever approach and techniques are chosen, the researcher must bear in mind the validity, reliability, and reactivity of the research methods finally applied.

VALIDITY

There are several different kinds and meanings of validity, but it is easiest to think of them as either *internal validity* or *external validity*.

Internal validity

This is about the measurement tools themselves. Are they measuring what you think they.are measuring? Are the data you are collecting a 'true' picture of what is happening? A good example of a test that lacked validity are the early intelligence tests. After some years of using these as an indication of the intellectual ability of children, it was realised that as the tests relied heavily on the meanings and relationships of words, they were really testing the pupils' understanding of the English language. Questionnaires can be more of a test of memory and the ability to recall events than a data collection method about a specific subject.

External validity

This concerns the appropriateness of the measurement tools to answer the research question. If you want to find out the feelings of a residents' association to a new community home for the mentally handicapped, would an attitude scale really show what they thought and, more importantly, how they would behave?

RELIABILITY

In research language, reliability refers to the extent to which the results would be the same if the data collection tools were re-applied at a different time, or in a different place. Reliability then is a factor on two levels: time and place.

First, if a questionnaire or other research tool was applied on a particular day, would the same result be obtained if the same method were applied at a later date to the same research sample?

Second, could the research tools be used with similar results in another place? If so, the findings of the research are applicable elsewhere.

Even seemingly tried and tested methods can lack reliability – how close is the agreement on a blood pressure reading taken by ten different nurses?

REACTIVITY

However carefully set up it is, all research – even an experiment – takes place in a social context. That is, people are required to interact with each other and with the setting and objects around them. So researcher and subjects will be reacting to each other's presence and behaviour. The extent to which this influences the research data is known as reactivity.

Suppose you were interviewed about your views on the wards you have worked on. Your answers might well be different if the questioner were one of the ward sisters than those you might give to someone unconnected with the hospital! It has been shown that people respond in a different way to male interviewers than to females.

Another way in which reactivity can occur is in the researcher's influence on the research situation itself or the data collected. In an interview for example, if the researcher appears shocked or ignores some things the respondent says, he or she will probably not mention these again. The researcher has, therefore, made some choices about what information is collected, and equally what is not, perhaps even without realising it. If the method being used involves the researcher as a participant, his or her actions will inevitably have some effect on the situation under study.

So far we have talked about choosing one research approach and one method. However there is another type of research design called triangulation.

You may have seen triangulation markers at the top of hills or other landmarks. These are obtained by taking sightings of the point from more than one direction, then marking where they meet. Triangulation in research means very much the same thing. The research question is tackled by different approaches, a variety of methods, even more than one theory. This serves two main purposes. First, it helps to confirm the results obtained by any one method. Second, by looking at the problem from another research approach, a different perspective can be brought to bear on the topic under investigation. Thus, the results can be treated with more confidence and a wider range of explanatory theory used and tested. Hopefully, greater illumination of the subject will be achieved.

Exercises

1. Write down all the research methods you can remember having heard about.
    Your list should include some of these:
    *   Questionnaires
    *   Interviews
    *   Observation
    *   Using records and documents
    *   Attitude scales

2. Imagine you are one of the case study team, Staff Nurse Baker for example. Decide what approach and method you feel would be most appropriate for the research you want to conduct. Then think of all the factors of validity, reliability and reactivity that must be considered and how they might be overcome. Having decided which research approach to use, the next question is what research technique or method would you choose to employ?

3. What are the differences between a nursing theory and a theory for nursing? In what kinds of research would each be relevant? Write down what you consider to be the important points here. If this is a class exercise, the question would provide an interesting discussion topic.

SCENARIO

Now let's return to our ward team and see what approach would be most suitable for them.

Sister Jones needs to look at the number of patients likely to be affected by the new policy. From this she will be able to deduce how this will change the work-load of her ward. One way of doing this would be to look at records of past operation lists. So her research will require a survey approach, and quantitative methods will provide the data she requires.

The community nurse, Sister Brown, is concerned about whether patients who are discharged from hospital soon after operation will take more time to care for at home. She realises that they will not only need specific nursing procedures such as dressings, but may also require counselling and teaching about their condition. They may be worried or their families may find it difficult to cope. A survey of patients referred will enable her to see how much community nursing time is taken up by patients after discharge, and, hopefully, give some indication of what time will be needed after the change of policy.

Sister Brown therefore decides to conduct a survey of patients referred over the next two months (which will give quantitative data). However, finding out how patients feel about being discharged fairly quickly from hospital will give her a better understanding of what extra demands may be made on her in the future by such patients. So Sister Brown will try also to develop a questionnaire for patients to gain their views. As data are to be sought from patients, the consent of the Ethical Committee will be necessary.

Staff Nurse Baker wishes to compare the ward's existing nursing process notes with an experimental set. In deciding how to go about this, the staff nurse must decide what questions she wants to answer. Does she want to know whether the experimental notes take longer to complete? If so, then structured non-participant observation would be appropriate in an open context. Or does she wish to see if nurses are able to use the new notes more easily to refer to in caring for patients, in which case, participant observation in a closed context might provide better data?

Alternatively, Staff Nurse Baker might be more concerned with the opinions of staff and patients about the new notes. These could best be sought in interviews, but she will have to find out how people feel about the old notes as well, otherwise how can she compare the two? Interviews will mean getting the permission of the Clinical Nurse Manager and, if patients are involved, the Ethical Committee. In the end Staff Nurse Baker decides that she wants to see if the new notes are easier to refer to in the day-to-day care of patients, so plans to set up an experimental situation using the old notes on one half of the ward and the new notes on the other.

Student Nurse Green plans to take the opportunity to carry out an assignment she has to complete using qualitative methods. As Staff Nurse Baker is planning to look at records, the student nurse decides to concentrate on patients and their attitudes. Her research will probably be interpretative in approach.

In each case, the members of the ward team have chosen the style that is the most appropriate for the questions they wish to answer. This, not methodological dogma, should always be the primary concern in any research.

BIBLIOGRAPHY

Birch J (1975) *To Nurse or not to Nurse.* London: Royal College of Nursing.

Bond S (1983) Nurses' communication with cancer patients. *Nursing Research, Ten Studies in Patient Care,* ed. J Wilson-Barnett, ch. 3. Chichester: John Wiley.

Carper B A (1978) Fundamental patterns of knowing in nursing. *Advances in Nursing Science,* **1** (1). In Ackerman W B and Lohnes P R, *Research Methods for Nurses.* New York: McGraw-Hill.

Cormack D F S (1984) Flanagan's critical incident technique. *The Research Process in Nursing,* ch. 12. Oxford: Blackwell Scientific Publications.

Duffy M E (1985) Designing nursing research: the qualitative–quantitative debate. *Journal of Advanced Nursing,* **10**: 225–232.

Field P A and Morse J M (1985) Approaches to theory development. *Nursing Research: The Application of Qualitative Approaches,* ch. 1. London and Sydney: Croom Helm.

Fox D J (1976) Research approaches. *Fundamentals of Research in Nursing,* ch. 9. New York: Appleton-Century-Crofts.

Glaser B and Strauss A (1967) *The Discovery of Grounded Theory: Strategies for Qualitative Research.* Chicago: Aldine Publishing Co.

Hockey L (1979) Indicators in nursing research with emphasis on social indicators. *Journal of Advanced Nursing,* **2** (3): 239–250.

Hockey L (1986) Nursing research: its pleasures, problems and potential for nursing. Paper presented at Wessex Regional Research Conference at Dorset Institute of Higher Education, Poole, 29 November 1986.

Macleod Clark J and Hockey L (1981) Overview of research design and methods. *Research for Nursing,* ch. 2. London: H M and M Publishers.

Macleod Clark J (1983) Nurse–patient communication: an analysis of conversations from surgical wards. *Nursing Research, Ten Studies in Patient Care,* ed. J Wilson-Barnett, ch. 2. Chichester: John Wiley.

McFarlane J (1977) Developing a theory of nursing: the relation of theory, practice, education and research. *Journal of Advanced Nursing,* **2** (3): 261–270.

Polit D and Hungler B (1985) Principles of research design. *Essentials of Nursing Research,* ch. 8. Philadelphia: J B Lippincott.

Rodin J (1983) Preparing children in hospital. *Nursing Research: Ten Studies in Patient Communication,* ed. J Wilson-Barnett, ch. 8. Chichester: John Wiley.

Seaman C H C and Verhonick P J (1982) Theory in nursing research. *Research Methods for Undergraduate Students in Nursing.* Norwalk, Conn.: Appleton-Century-Crofts.

Towell D (1975) *Understanding Psychiatric Nursing: A Sociological Study of Modern Psychiatric Nursing Practice.* London: Royal College of Nursing.

Treece E W and Treece J W (1986) Reliability and validity. *Elements of Research in Nursing,* ch. 15. St Louis: C V Mosby.

UKCC Project 2000 Project Paper 8 (1987) London: United Kingdom Central Council for Nursing, Midwifery and Health Visiting.

Webb C (1983) A study of recovery from hysterectomy. *Nursing Research: Ten Studies in Patient Care,* ed. J Wilson-Barnett, ch. 10. Chichester: John Wiley.

Weiss C H (ed.) (1977) *Using Social Research in Public Policy Making.* Mass.: Lexington Books.

Wells T (1979) *Problems in Geriatric Care: A Study of Nurses' Problems in Care of Old People in Hospitals.* Edinburgh: Churchill Livingstone.

6

Experimental Methods

Like Staff Nurse Baker in our scenario, you might decide on an experimental approach for your research study because it offers the possibility of establishing links between change and its consequences with 'hard' quantitative data. Experimental methods are all about finding causal connections, usually through comparison of different groups or states, by following strict logical rules. We can be reasonably confident about the results because measurements are made under controlled conditions. The results can be helpful in understanding why things happen and predicting future events. Statistical tests have been designed to check whether any differences shown in the results are due to our intervention or just chance (see Chapter 10 on analysing data).

We should remember, however, that numbers can give a false sense of security. Unless we are studying under strict laboratory conditions there will always be some doubt about the variability of measurements, especially if the study is of variable, fallible human beings in natural surroundings!

In the last chapter we described the three main styles of experiment, survey and interpretative research. We have chosen to start with experiments in this chapter, continuing our discussion of which methods to choose in research design. This is not because we are particularly recommending experimental design, as all methods have a value in answering research questions. It really depends on the question. We are starting with the experiment because it is at one end of the continuum of methods deriving from different theoretical perspectives in nursing, the most structured and quantitative end. It represents the purest form of scientific enquiry discussed in Chapter 1. In the following chapters we will cover the main styles in turn, so that they can be compared with each other, until we reach the other end of the continuum, the qualitative methods, which represent a reaction to the scientific tradition.

DEFINITIONS

Experimental methods are quite familiar at an everyday level, in the idea of the classic 'before and after' design and in health care as the basis for much medical research, such as drug trials. The method is used in nursing research, as for example the classic studies by Hayward (1975) and Boore (1978), where patients' responses to pain, after pre-operative information, were compared with those receiving routine treatment. The principles of experimental design are also applied in evaluation and action research so current in the climate of quality assurance in the health services today, and will be dealt with later in the chapter.

Let us try to define the experiment precisely to see how it can be applied to solve problems in nursing practice. Colin Robson gives a nice straightforward definition in his book, *Design and Statistics in Psychology* (1973):

> In an experiment, one investigates the relationship between two (or more) things by deliberately producing a change in one of them and looking at, observing the change in the other. These 'things' in which change takes place are usually called variables.

The word variable simply means something that can vary – a characteristic of a person or object that varies, can be observed, and can be measured.

Experiments are, therefore, very relevant to assessing changes in nursing practice and nursing services generally. If a new medication for pressure sores were introduced, for instance, we would be interested to see if the rate of healing varied compared to other treatments. Experimental design could help us to do this accurately. At another level, experimental design has been used to compare the quality of life of residents in a long-stay hospital with those in new community units. In the scenario, Staff Nurse Baker intends to compare the effects on patients of two different approaches to the nursing process.

The convention for studying variables in experiments is to identify them as independent and dependent variables. The *independent variable* is the one that we manipulate deliberately to produce change. In our example above the treatment for pressure sores is the independent variable. In the case of the comparison of hospital and community care, the independent variable is the model of care.

It follows that the *dependent* variable is the one we look at for change.

Exercise

Can you identify the dependent variable in each of our two examples and suggest how they could be measured?

Discussion

In the first example the condition of the pressure sores is our dependent variable whereas in the second it is the quality of life of the residents. There are a variety of ways in which the dependent variables could be measured. The effect of medication on the pressure sores could be measured by the speed of healing in terms of time, by changes in their size or by any other observable signs. Suggestions for measuring the quality of life of long-stay residents might include the range and number of daily activities, contacts with the community, number of visitors or their own opinions.

Now that we have begun to explore what experimental design means we can develop the ideas by examining some more complex definitions of experiments. An Open University course on social research methods defines the experiment as:

> measurement under conditions of systematic control of different features of the research setting. (Open University, 1984)

A Dictionary of Social Science Methods says:

> A study undertaken to test one or more hypotheses and in which the relevant variables are controlled and manipulated by the experimenter, rather than simply observed in their natural setting. (Miller and Wilson, 1983)

These quotations introduce two further points: that experiments follow from hypotheses and the question of control of variables. A further consideration is that of ethics when applying principles of experimental design to human individuals. We shall be dealing with these points in the following sections.

HYPOTHESES

We mentioned hypotheses in the first and second chapters. An hypothesis offers a possible explanation for a research problem. Sometimes it is simply stated as a question. The point about a hypothesis is that it is a clear statement of the likely outcome of an experiment, which the research will either support or reject. The rejection of the hypothesis is also anticipated at the outset and expressed as a 'null hypothesis'. This is a convention in statistical testing of results that will be explained in more detail later and in Chapter 10. To take one of our earlier examples, the hypothesis might be:

> Residents in a community home have more contacts with their relatives than residents in a long-stay hospital.

Whereas the *null* hypothesis would say:

> Residents in a community home have no more contacts with their relatives than residents in a long-stay hospital.

In the scientific approach, writing an hypothesis is the next stage after the initial statement of the research problem and a review of the literature. It is central to theory building where every new idea is tested rigorously to add to our knowledge about the world and in turn stimulates further investigation. The hypothesis should predict the relationship between the independent and dependent variables of interest in a way that can be measured. The statement of the problem needs to be successively refined and narrowed, therefore, so that the focus is on the main variables, how they can be researched and the likely outcome of their association or the effect of changes in one on the other. This may generate more than one hypothesis. If we take the example from Chapter 2, where we arrived at the statement of a problem as:

> Can non-verbal communication be used effectively by nurses as a means of initiating leisure activities with adults with a profound mental handicap in a residential setting?

we could express this in the form of at least four separate hypotheses for testing:

1. Nurses vary in their use of non-verbal skills with clients.
2. The greater the use of non-verbal skills by nurses, the more effective they are in initiating activities with clients.
3. Clients will vary in their responsiveness to non-verbal skills.
4. Training staff in the use of non-verbal skills will increase their effectiveness with clients in initiating activities.

The literature review helps in the refining of a problem statement into a hypothesis and this is why one should continue reading parallel to the design stages of a research study.

The exploratory stages of a study will also assist in how to convert or operationalise ideas in the statement into observable, measurable variables. In our example of the pressure sores we showed that various measures could be used to indicate the effectiveness of medication.

A good hypothesis, therefore, will suggest the design for a research study that would attempt to prove or disprove its predictions. Hypotheses allow for the possibility that there will be no effect between the independent variable and the dependent variable. Statistical tests used with experimental data are based on the principle of the 'null hypothesis' – that there is no relationship expected between the variables – so if their measurement does show a related variation that is taken as a significant result.

We cannot really talk about 'proof' in such absolute terms, however. Results of experimental studies are usually worded more tentatively, talking of how results 'support' or 'tend to confirm' the hypothesis.

CONTROL OF VARIABLES

If a tutor wanted to try a different way of teaching, say exercises rather than lectures as the means of teaching research methods, how could the results of the new approach be evaluated? First, if the new approach were to be checked in a fairly scientific way, a hypothesis would be needed. For example:

> Exercises are a more successful way of teaching research methods to nursing students than lectures.

The simplest evaluation would be a type of case study where the results of the group learning by the new approach could be measured in some way. This can be represented in diagrammatic form as in Figure 6.1.

Independent variable (IV)	Dependent variable (DV)
Teaching research by exercises	Group's response

Time ——————————————➤

Figure 6.1 Simple design for measuring effects of the independent variable

The independent variable is the new teaching approach but could represent any intervention or change. The dependent variable here is the effect on the group of students.

Exercise

How could the dependent variable be operationalised and measured in this example?

Discussion

Various measures could be used to assess the success of different teaching approaches. The conventional means, of course, are exams and assignments to test students' knowledge on remembered facts. Other methods could include asking the students to rate the new approach, seeing how much time it took to cover the topics or simply counting how many students fell asleep!

Exercise

Can you see any problems with the case study method as an experimental design?

Discussion

You might have mentioned that it would be more sensible to compare the effects of the *two* teaching approaches, which would look something like Figure 6.2 in diagrammatic form:

IV	DV
Lectures	Group's response
Exercises	Group's response

Time ─────────────────────→

Figure 6.2 Design for comparing two versions of the independent variable

DV	IV	DV
Group's knowledge	Teaching approach	Group's knowledge

Time ─────────────────────→

Figure 6.3 Design for measuring before and after the introduction of the independent variable

Sometimes, it is possible to try two different types of intervention on the same group and compare the results. In our example it might be all right to compare teaching by lectures or exercises with the same group if we were measuring something like students' alertness or sleepiness. But if we wanted to check *learning* on a specific topic, we would have to use two groups – a different group for each of the two methods. Otherwise the learning from whichever method was used to start with would affect the learning from the method which followed. In this case it would be vital to match the two groups so that they were similar in most respects, to be sure that any differences in student performance were due to the different teaching approaches.

Another important point might be what the group or groups were like beforehand. If we were checking something such as knowledge, this would need to be assessed before and after the intervention of the independent variable (the teaching approach) (Figure 6.3).

EXPERIMENTAL DESIGN

Combining the two considerations we arrive at the classic experimental before-and-after design with an experimental group and a control group (Figure 6.4).

DV	IV	DV
Control group's response	Lectures	Control group's response
Experimental group's response	Exercises	Experimental group's response

Time ————————————➤

Figure 6.4 Before and after design with control group for comparison

With this design we can more confidently compare differences in performance (whatever the measure used) to see if they support the hypothesis that teaching research methods by exercises is a more effective approach.

More complex designs can be used with more than two groups or with several controlled dependent and independent variables.

Exercise

In our example of the tutor teaching research methods, can you see any other problems in comparing the two different teaching groups?

Discussion

As we have already observed, there may be factors other than the indentified independent variable that could influence the outcome of the different teaching approaches.

Even if the groups were matched as far as possible in terms of age, sex, race, ability, etc. there might be differences in the conditions in which the classes took place. Did the classes happen in the same place, the same room? Did they have the same teacher? If the groups were taught in different years or on different days, were there other events happening that might have made a difference? For instance, in one year a gloomy economic or political mood may exist as a backdrop to all activities. Fridays might have a different atmosphere from Mondays. Timing is obviously important too. The events such as other lessons that precede the research teaching might influence students' receptiveness. If we are using the number of students who fall asleep as an indicator, lessons after lunch are notoriously soporific!

If the student group were more sleepy in a lecture session after lunch than the other group in a morning session of exercises, we could not necessarily conclude that the lecture was less successful because there are other variables such as time of day operating as competing independent variables. These are called uncontrolled, extraneous or confounding variables. The only way to achieve a true comparison would be to compare two different teaching sessions under as similar conditions as possible. It would be interesting to compare two post-lunch sessions, for example, to see if fewer people fell asleep in the exercise session as hypothesised.

Our example here has demonstrated what was meant in the earlier definition of the experiment as 'systematic control of different features of the research setting' and 'relevant variables are controlled and manipulated by the experimenter'. Unless potentially confounding variables are controlled they could systematically bias the results, so that in manipulating the independent variable, the experimenter may inadvertently manipulate other things at the same time. We need to be sure that the effects on the dependent variable are due to the chosen independent variable. There can be problems with the measurement of the dependent variable, too, and particular attention needs to be paid to the validity and reliability of the measures, as discussed in the previous chapter.

Control of variables is critical if one is looking for causal connections between the variables. The rules for establishing causality are:

1. There must be evidence of an association between the independent variable/s and the dependent variable/s (conventionally called X and Y).
2. X must be prior in time to Y.
3. No other variable can explain the effects on Y, otherwise the effect could be called 'spurious'. The association between smoking and lung cancer has also been called spurious because both could be caused by other psycho-physical factors.

SUMMARY

We conclude this section with a summary of the discussion on the logic and definitions of experiments:

1. In the most basic form of the experiment, a chosen group is given an experimental treatment that is systematically controlled.
2. A control group, which is chosen in the same way from the same population, does not receive the experimental treatment, but all other conditions are the same.
3. The treatment that is changed is called the independent variable.
4. Both groups are assessed on some outcome measure that is the dependent variable.
5. If the groups differ on the dependent variable, the conclusion is that the change in the independent variable had caused the difference and the hypothesis is confirmed.
6. Alternative explanations for the differences are controlled for by ensuring that the groups are equivalent in all respects except for the one being tested.

QUASI-EXPERIMENTS

Although the classic before-and-after design shown in Figure 6.4 (above) is the ideal for experiments, the other designs illustrated are also viable and may often be the only option in natural settings. It is here that experiment becomes more quasi-experiment. For instance, there may only be data available for one group or the only groups that can be compared have not been matched. Cook and Campbell's book on quasi-experimentation (1979) provides some useful statistical tactics to compensate for the lack of rigour in design.

ETHICS

The appeal of experimental methods, as we have seen, is their potential to determine facts and links between them. Most of us experience serious reservations, however, about the application of experimental methods to people. Experiments on rats, for example, show a link between smoking and cancer, but this cannot ethically be replicated with human subjects. Some would say that the methods were unethical with animals too.

The rigour of experimental control can clash with social and professional values such as care and concern for the individual, maintenance and preservation of life. It is not ethical, for instance, for a nurse to withhold treatment from a group just for the sake of comparing that group with another. We cannot make patients or clients suffer in the name of research.

The ethical issues surrounding research are examined more fully in Chapter 9. We want here to quote some examples of experimental research in nursing where the researcher may have had to compromise on scientific rigour to keep within professional codes of conduct. Most such studies compare a new intervention with the existing one or offer different interventions to each group rather than deny the control group treatment. In an experimental study of touch by midwives to alleviate anxiety in labour (Lorenson, 1983), for instance, the control group were still given routine treatment. Some dubious practices still exist, however. In a comparison of family-planning methods, the difference between groups was measured by unplanned pregnancies! Now, whereas the volunteers were said to be willing, it does seem unethical to ask a group to try a contraceptive with unknown risks, and possible long-term effects on their lives.

The medical profession has helped to establish some ground rules through its tradition of drug trials research, and all proposed health-service research involving patients must now be submitted to a local committee for scrutiny. The operation of ethical committees is again discussed in more detail in the next chapter.

Exercise

For years it has been an advertising ploy to say that people can't tell the difference between margarine and butter, that a certain fizzy drink 'is it', a new additive in toothpaste is better at fighting decay, that one washing powder washes brighter and cleaner than the rest, that one brand of washing-up liquid washes more dishes, etc.

This exercise is to help you design an experiment to see if one brand of washing-up liquid really does wash more dishes. Once you have designed it you can actually try it out, if you like, to perfect the design and check the hypothesis.

Question
We'll start with the *hypothesis*. How would you word it?

Answer
You probably thought of something like:

Liquid detergent A will wash more dishes than liquid detergent B.

The *null* hypothesis would be that:

There will be no difference in the number of dishes washed by liquid detergent A compared with liquid detergent B.

Question

Which is the independent and which the dependent variable?

Answer

Washing-up liquids are the independent variable, whereas number of dishes washed is the dependent variable.

Question

How could the dependent variable be measured?

Answer

You could see whether a bottle of liquid detergent A lasted longer than a bottle of liquid detergent B – say between two families or in the same family trying one bottle after the other. Of course, you would have to check that the bottles were of the same size and that the amount of washing up averaged about the same in both cases. These are possible confounding variables that would have to be controlled.

A quicker way of comparing the two liquids that you have probably already thought of is to see how many dishes one measure of liquid detergent A can wash in one session compared with an equivalent measure of liquid detergent B. The hypothesis could be refined further to:

Liquid detergent A will wash more dishes in one session than the same measure of liquid detergent B.

This should be an easier situation to control accurately.

Question

What factors could act as confounding variables and should be controlled for?

Answer

1. Ideally the same person (yourself?) should conduct both trials.

2. The same measure must be used for both liquids.
3. The bowl and implements, cloths, etc. must be similar.
4. The water temperature should be similar.
5. The detergent should be added to the water at the same point.
6. The amount of agitation given to the detergent in the water should be the same.
7. The degree of greasiness of the dishes should not vary too much between trials.
8. The point at which you judge how many dishes have been washed will have to be fixed. Is it when the bubbles disappear from the dishwater or when the dishes no longer look clean (and what is the criterion for 'clean')?

You may have thought of other considerations and more would probably emerge when you put it to the test. Differences in skin temperature or cleanliness might have an effect, for instance. In this case it would be better to use rubber gloves for all trials, cleaning them in the same way between trials.

The order in which you tried the different washing up liquids might have an influence. One way round this in experimental design is to conduct more than one trial of each liquid deciding the order randomly by the toss of a coin and making sure conditions were as similar as possible at the beginning of each trial.

In Chapter 10 on data analysis we will see how results from an experiment like this could be fed into a statistical formula to test for significant results. That means we could test whether the results supported the experimental hypothesis or the null hypothesis – are any differences in the measures due to a real difference between the two products or have the differences occurred purely by chance?

EVALUATION AND ACTION RESEARCH

This section explores the application of experimental or quasi-experimental methods to the evaluation of practice and services. The following imaginary little piece of dialogue characterises the current trend for accountability in the health services today (Mager, 1968):

'You can't measure the effects of what I do.'
  'Why not?'
'They're intangible.'
  'Oh? Why should I pay you for intangible results?'
'Because I've been trained and licensed to practise.'
  'Hmm . . . all right. Here's your money.'
'Where? I don't see it.'
  'Of course not . . . it's intangible.'

All health professionals are now being asked to set standards and measure the effects of what they are doing. Cost-effectiveness does not, however, have to mean the sacrifice of quality of care. Evaluation research is well suited to this task, yielding useful data for practitioners and service planners. The methods have been developed since the Second World War, especially in the United States, in industry and human services where there is a need to justify costs for continued funding.

Information on national and international perspectives on evaluation research in health care can be obtained from: The Quality Assurance Information Service (QAIS), King's Fund Centre, 126 Albert Street, London NW1 7NF (Tel. 01-267 6111).

Evaluation methods adopt the classic experimental design because it promises a way of systematically assessing change in services. There are the difficulties of applying experiments in natural settings, of course, with associated problems of validity. As it is applied research, other methods are often used within a broad experimental framework. Thus in Lathlean and Farrish's (1984) study of ward sisters a survey was used for the evaluation. Even qualitative methods such as unstructured interviews and observation have been used to collect data in an experimental design. For example, in Smith and Cantley's (1985) study of a new day hospital for ESMI patients they interviewed staff and patients to determine the criteria for the success of the service. Unstructured observation was used in a similar study in an ESMI ward in Blandford (Couchman and Bradshaw, 1987). The mix of social science research methods is easily justified by reference to the argument for triangulation, discussed in the last chapter as a means of strengthening the validity of results.

To define 'evaluation research' we must distinguish it from the everyday usage of the word 'evaluation'. Luker (1981) points out that in everyday nursing evaluation simply means judgment. Evaluation research demands a more systematic or scientific collection of information about people, performance or products in order to improve effectiveness.

Evaluation is designed to answer the questions 'How are we doing?' and 'Are we achieving our goals?' – the effect of a new policy on nurse performance for example. Weiss (1972) called it a comparison of 'What is' with 'What should be'. It follows a process of:

Planning ⟶ Action ⟶ Evaluation

which corresponds to the problem-solving models we mentioned in the introductory chapters and to the experimental format:

1. A problem is stated.
2. An hypothesis is formulated for testing (i.e. a possible explanation is suggested).
3. Facts are gathered from observation or experimentation.

4. These facts are interpreted to see if the hypothesis was right.
5. Conclusions are drawn about solutions to the problem.

Evaluation, like experimental research, is concerned, therefore, with before-and-after measures, comparing groups, the relationship between variables, and controls. Our earlier example of the comparison of a community unit and traditional hospital illustrates the approach well.

The terms evaluation research and action research are often used interchangeably, but evaluation research is more the measurement of past changes whereas action research incorporates the change or intervention into the study. The researcher, in fact, becomes the agent of change. It is more the comparison of 'What is' with 'What could be'. The process of Planning → Action → Evaluation is perhaps better viewed as a cycle where the evaluation stage, in turn, generates ideas for further planning and action. With more detail of the tasks and skills involved this would look like Figure 6.5:

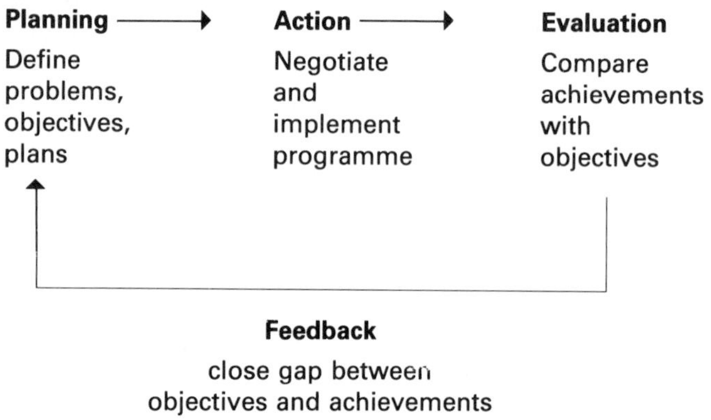

Planning ⟶   **Action** ⟶   **Evaluation**

Define   Negotiate   Compare
problems,   and   achievements
objectives,   implement   with
plans   programme   objectives

Feedback
close gap between
objectives and achievements

Figure 6.5 The evaluation cycle

Remember the poem by Mager (1968) in Chapter 2? The last verse went like this:

To rise from a zero
To Big Nursing Hero
To answer these questions you'll strive:
    Where am I going,
    How shall I get there, and
    How will I know I've arrived?

In other words:

If you don't know where you're going, how can you tell when you've got there?

Santaya, a philosopher said:

Those who don't learn from history are doomed to repeat it.

The difficulty in an evaluation study is finding the right indicators to measure, as in any quantitative study. Patton, who has written several imaginative books about evaluation says:

Few things evade our attention so consistently as those things we take for granted. (Patton, 1981)

Perhaps, then, in evaluating services or practice we are helping people to recognise what they already know but have not made conscious?

Karen Luker (1981) has likened evaluation research to the stages of:

Structure → Process → Outcome

in systems theory. This helps to highlight the fact that, although outcomes are important, we might need to take account of other variables – the 'means' as well as the 'ends'. The kind of factors you might consider in a nursing study could be:

1. *Structure*: facilities, equipment, staffing, style of management.
2. *Process*: forms of care.
3. *Outcome*: whether patients' objectives have been met.

Again, as Luker points out, this model coincides with the nursing process. The actual choice of variables would depend on the circumstances and purposes of the study.

Exercise

Imagine that I have to buy a house for you. List the factors that you would want me to remember when selecting a suitable house. Ask other people you know to do the exercise and compare lists.

Discussion

The important point about this exercise is that whereas there would be some common factors on your lists, there would also be a lot of differences. Different people have different perspectives on what would be a successful outcome and the same applies to evaluation research.

Smith and Cantley's (1985) study of the ESMI day hospital was interesting in that they aimed at a 'pluralistic' evaluation to represent the views of the different groups involved (and to triangulate results). In interviews with staff and families they revealed quite contradictory criteria for the success of the service. The staff perceived the carers' support group, for instance, as providing relief to families and preventing admission to long-term care and assumed that the service should be evaluated in those terms. The majority of carers, on the other hand, said when interviewed that they only attended the support group in an attempt to persuade the staff to admit their relative to care!

Greenwood (1984) has suggested that action research is the only relevant research method for a practical discipline such as nursing. We would remind you, however, of the argument in Chapter 5. There is a danger in this kind of research, where the problems are defined by policy-makers within unquestioned frameworks of knowledge. Smith and Cantley (1985) believe that researchers do not have to solve problems in the way they are expected to if they can demonstrate convincingly that the problem is best formulated another way. Perhaps the theory and value bases need to be made explicit at the outset. It is useful sometimes to identify whether the research is intended to meet the needs of the client or the service, because the ideas of the researcher and those who commissioned the research can be at odds.

If nurses are to become involved in evaluation, they must enter into a dialogue as professionals developing their own theories and values of care. Evaluation can be 'formative' (Morris and Fitz-Gibbon, 1978; Burton, 1986) so that the researcher plays an interactive role in the collecting and sharing of information with practitioners and planners during the development of a programme of care.

This particular approach can be helpful in overcoming any resistance from practitioners in the work setting. The idea of an outsider coming in to evaluate can be very threatening. If people are involved in the research they are more likely to use the results.

Patton (1982) calls it a 'Collaborative Evaluation' model. It is a team effort with team members representing different groups or disciplines who have a 'stake' in the outcome (Patton describes them as 'stake-holders'). The model was used in the Blandford study quoted earlier (Couchman and Bradshaw, 1987) and in other studies in the mental health field (Towell and Harries, 1979; Evans and Blunden, 1984).

The last words should go to Patton (1981) who reminds us not to take evaluation too seriously:

Him to her
Evaluators make better lovers because they are constantly assessing their performance to improve it.

Her to him
Being aware of a thing and being able to do something about it are two quite different things!

SCENARIO

In this chapter you have experienced experimental design in some light-hearted exercises. Now we would like you to apply your emerging skills to the design of Staff Nurse Baker's project, which is more like an evaluation/action research style.

If you remember, in the last chapter she had decided to compare the ease of reference to new nursing process notes on one half of the ward with the use of the existing notes on the other half.

Exercise

This exercise can be done on an individual basis or adapted to group discussion.

Following similar steps to the washing-up liquid experiment, try answering the following questions to help you design the study.

- Is it a classic experimental design?
- What other methods could be used?
- How should the subjects be chosen?
- How many are needed?
- What would be the hypothesis?
- What are the independent and dependent variables?
- What measures could be used?
- Could they be valid and reliable?
- What are the possible confounding variables to control for?
- Can you satisfy the rules of causality?
- Could you generalise the results to other groups?
- Is the design ethically sound?

Discussion

Compare your design with the one arrived at by Staff Nurse Baker.

The first task was to decide how to measure 'ease of reference' to the new nursing notes. Staff Nurse Baker considered various options. She could observe how frequently staff actually referred to the notes but that could be very time consuming for a 'part-time researcher' like herself, even if she only observed for sample times of the day. She did wonder about narrowing the focus of observation to the number of times nurses were seen to refer to the notes during ward rounds, but that was still quite a time commitment.

She considered a survey or interviews with staff for their opinions of the different methods but felt that might be rather subjective. Some of the issues about subjectivity and objectivity were raised in Chapter 5 and will be discussed further in Chapter 8 on qualitative methods.

In the end, Staff Nurse Baker chose to use measures from the nursing process notes themselves, such as how many goals were set and achieved for patients and changes to the notes based on evaluation. She judged these to be reasonably valid indicators, according to the various criteria. She asked a tutor to cross-check a sample of results for reliability (validity and reliability are dealt with in Chapter 5).

The hypothesis for the study was therefore:

'The new nursing process notes will make it easier for nurses to keep notes up to date.'

The independent variable was the introduction of the new system for notes and the dependent variable the frequency of additions to the notes.

The comparison of one half of the ward with the other has an experimental design like Figure 6.2. The half with the new nursing process notes are the experimental group (A), and the half using existing notes are the control group (B) (Figure 6.6):

IV	DV
New notes	Group A
Existing notes	Group B

Time ──────────────────➤

Figure 6.6   Comparison design

An alternative would have been a before-and-after design on the same group (Figure 6.7):

DV	IV	DV
Group before change	New notes	Group after change

Time ──────────────────➤

Figure 6.7   Before-and-after design

Indeed, Staff Nurse Baker could have combined the two approaches in a classic experimental design, where she measured groups A and B before and after the introduction of new nursing process notes with group A. She decided to keep the design as simple as possible, however, because of the variability in the setting.

The simplest way of deciding who was in which group was to start by 'matching pairs' – choosing a pair of men or women who matched roughly on several important characteristics such as age or condition – and then randomly selecting one for group A by the toss of a coin. In this way she was controlling for confounding or competing independent variables. It was also the most ethical procedure, although the people in group B would not be denied treatment, as they were being nursed under the old regime.

Of course, Staff Nurse Baker was aware that with only 12 in each group on the ward at any one time she would not be able to make statistical comparisons or generalise findings to other groups. She proposed to refine her design with the initial groups, and then study incoming patients over several weeks, each new patient being randomly allocated to the groups, until she had data on 30 patients in each group.

BIBLIOGRAPHY

Boore J (1978) *A Prescription for Recovery*. London: Royal College of Nursing.
Burton M (1986) What do we mean by evaluation? *Health Service Journal*, 17 July, pp.954–955.
Cook T D and Campbell D T (1979) *Quasi-experimentation: Design and Analysis Issues for Field Studies*. Chicago: Rand McNally.
Cormack D F S (ed.) (1984) *The Research Process in Nursing*, chs 10 and 13. Oxford: Blackwell.
Couchman W and Bradshaw P (1987). A measure of the lifestyles of two groups of elderly mentally ill people. Paper presented at 'In Pursuit of Excellence' Conference, London, 2 November 1987.
Evans G and Blunden R (1984) A collaborative approach to evaluation. *Journal of Practical Approaches to Developmental Handicap*, **8** (1): 14–18.
Greenwood J (1984) Nursing research: a position paper. *Journal of Advanced Nursing*, **9** (1): 77–82.
Hayward J (1975) *Information: a Prescription Against Pain*. London: Royal College of Nursing.
Lathlean J and Farrish S (1984) *The Ward Sister Training Project: An Evaluation of a Training Scheme for Ward Sisters*. London: DHSS.
Lorenson M (1983) Effects of touch in patients during a crisis situation in hospital. *Nursing Research: Ten Studies in Patient Care*, ed. Wilson-Barnett J, ch 9. Chichester: John Wiley and Sons.
Luker K (1981) An overview of evaluation research in nursing. *Journal of Advanced Nursing*, **6**: 87–93.
Mager R F (1968) *Developing Attitude Toward Learning*. California: Fearon Pitman Publishers.
Miller S (1975) *Experimental Design and Statistics*. London: Methuen.
Miller P McC and Wilson M J (1983) *A Dictionary of Social Science Methods*. Chichester: John Wiley and Sons.
Morris L L and Fitz-Gibbon C T (1978). *Program Evaluation Kit*. London: Sage Publications.

Open University (1984) *Research Methods in Education and the Social Sciences.* Milton Keynes: Open University Press.

Patton M Q (1981) *Creative Evaluation.* London: Sage Publications.

Patton M Q (1982) *Practical Evaluation.* London: Sage Publications.

Polit D and Hungler B (1983) *Nursing Research: Principles and Method,* ch. 6. Philadelphia: J B Lippincott.

Robson C (1973) *Experiment, Design and Statistics in Psychology.* Harmondsworth: Penguin Books.

Smith G and Cantley C (1985) Policy evaluation: the use of varied data in a study of a psychogeriatric service. *Applied Qualitative Research,* ed. R Walker, pp.156–174. London: Gower.

Treece E W and Treece J W (1977) *Elements of Research in Nursing.* New York: C V Mosby.

Towell D and Harries C (1979) *Innovation in Patient Care.* London: Croom Helm.

Weiss C H (1972) *Evaluation Research: Methods for Assessing Program Effectiveness.* Englewood Cliffs, N.J.: Prentice-Hall.

7

Survey Methods

In our scenario, Sister Brown will be using surveys to assess the demands on the community nurse of early discharge and to find out the feelings of patients and carers. She now needs to find out more about conducting a survey.

The survey is probably the research method that we are all most familiar with. Almost all of us at some time will have been stopped in the street for a market research survey of our opinions of some biscuits or domestic cleaner or other. There is also the census, of course, which is a survey on a massive scale involving everyone in the country. You may also have taken part in a survey at work by completing a questionnaire on, say, back pain or testing a new product or procedure.

Because it is such a familiar method, many people who want to do a research project feel that they must do a survey when, as we pointed out in Chapter 5 on research design, there is a range of methods from which to choose. It is important to start with your research question and then find the best method to address it, rather than finding a question to fit the method.

Familiarity with the method can also breed contempt. Some people seem to believe that, like writing a novel, designing a questionnaire is something that anyone can do without any kind of training. This shows, unfortunately, in quite a lot of questionnaires that are used in research and the researcher is doomed to learn from his or her mistakes. Questions are asked in ways that will produce invalid or meaningless responses. A few simple guidelines can help to avoid wasted time and effort.

DEFINITION

A survey, as we defined it in Chapter 5, is:

> The use of questionnaires, tests and interviews with large samples of the population.

Surveys are more 'open-ended' than experimental methods. Whereas an experiment seeks to *explain* the relationship between variables according to a prediction or hypothesis, the survey more often *describes* what has been found out about the characteristics studied and their relationships.

SURVEY STYLES

There are two basic means of data collection in surveys:

1.   the postal or self-completion quesionnaire
2.   the interview

although the same rules of design generally apply to both. Which type you choose will depend on certain constraints such as cost.

The self-completion type is relatively cheap, even if postage is involved. Instructions for completion must, however, be very clear and precise.

Interviews can be very time-consuming and interviewers may need to be paid. There are problems about consistency of style if more than one interviewer is used. Characteristics of the interviewer may influence the respondents, if they are of a different age, gender or class. On the other hand, face-to-face interaction can be a great advantage because the interviewer has the opportunity to probe certain areas in more depth.

Just as there is a continuum of research methods from the most to the least structured, so survey styles vary by degree of structure. At one end of the scale is the large survey with a structured questionnaire or interview schedule. At the other end of the scale is the unstructured interview. In between are various semi-structured formats for questionnaires and interviews. 'Structure' refers to the degree of standardisation or focus in the questions. Figure 7.1 shows a structured questionnaire with standard questions – everybody is asked the same questions, in the same way and in the same order, so that variations in the responses can be compared.

Figure 7.2 is an example of a structured interview. Even though the questions are open they are still the same, or standard, for every respondent.

The interview guide in Figure 7.3 is semi-structured because, whereas there is some structure or focus provided by the headings, the ordering and asking of the questions is flexible.

Unstructured interviews are more like conversations. The interviewer will start with some broad topics but will allow the interviewee to talk freely. This style is rarely used in survey research, except perhaps in the early stages, and is discussed more fully in Chapter 8 on qualitative techniques.

The question of how structured your questionnaire should be depends very much on the purpose of the research. If your area of research is fairly exploratory, where you are trying to find out something about a little known

WHERE ARE YOU NOW?   *Office*

If you are a part-time nursing degree graduate we would be   *use*
grateful if you could answer the following questions:

1. In which area was your career *before* the degree?
    (Please tick one box)
    Clinical/Community   ☐
    Education   ☐
    Management   ☐
    Other   ☐
    (if 'Other' please specify)

    ....

2. In which area was your career *during* the degree?
    (Please tick one box)
    Clinical/Community   ☐
    Education   ☐
    Management   ☐
    Other   ☐
    (if 'Other' please specify)

    ....

3. In which area was your career *after* the degree?
    (Please tick one box)
    Clinical/Community   ☐
    Education   ☐
    Management   ☐
    Other   ☐
    (if 'Other' please specify)

    ....

4. Are you . . .
    (Tick one box)
    Female?   ☐
    Male?   ☐

5. Do you have any other comments?
    (Please write overleaf)

MANY THANKS FOR YOUR HELP

Figure 7.1   An example of a structured questionnaire

READING HABITS SURVEY

1. Which nursing journals do you read?

2. Do you buy any nursing journals?
   (If YES, which ones?)

3. When do you read journals (at work, at home, etc.)?

4. Which topics do you like to read about?

5. How far away is your nearest hospital library?

6. When did you last visit a hospital library?

Thanks for your help

Figure 7.2   An example of a structured interview schedule

area, a very structured format might impose too many constraints and a semi-structured or unstructured format would be more appropriate.

VIEWS ON NURSING PROCESS – INTERVIEW GUIDE

(Ask the questions in your own words, and in a different order if appropriate. Probe as necessary.)

Introduction
Introduce self as student doing course.
Explain that doing study as project on views of qualified nurses about the nursing process.
Stress confidentiality.

Main questions
1. Does the nurse use the nursing process?
2. If used, how is it used?
3. Definition of nursing process?
4. How learned/trained about nursing process?
5. Level of commitment to nursing process?
6. Statement of pros and cons?

Background details
Age
Speciality
Year qualified
Postbasic qualifications

(Thank interviewee.)

Figure 7.3   An example of a semi-structured interview guide

Structured questionnaires or interview schedules such as those shown in Figures 7.1 and 7.2 are the ideal method for obtaining information from large numbers of people. They can be used to gain data on attitudes, beliefs and opinions from a wide range of people, relatively quickly and cheaply.

The data lend themselves to statistical analysis to show large-scale social patterns and trends. It follows that the style is best used for numbers about a hundred and above, and in an area where the boundaries for research are already quite well established.

Many nursing studies have successfully taken this approach. Structured surveys have been used to assess nurses' attitudes towards their role, their practice and their training and towards specific groups of patients. Patients have been asked for their opinions on their care before admission, and before and after leaving hospital. Clark and Hockey (1979, 1988) provide a useful summary of many of these studies.

On the other side of the coin, the disadvantages of the structured method are that it can be a bit too broad, general and superficial. There is also the vexed question of validity. How can you be sure that your questions mean the same to everybody and will elicit accurate information on the subject you are interested in? Sometimes it feels as if the respondents are being pigeonholed, or forced into artificial categories. The other major problem is the 'words/deeds dilemma' – people will say one thing and do another. For example, a respondent might be able to tell you all about the importance of exercise for health and in reality lead a very sedentary life. Most of the guidelines on the design of questionnaires exist to try and tackle this problem and we have given some useful references at the end of this chapter.

PROCEDURE

There are three main stages in constructing a structured questionnaire for a survey.

1. Exploratory stage.
2. Pilot study.
3. Main survey.

Stages 1 and 2 are very important in order to overcome some of the problems in the main survey that we have discussed.

Exploratory stage

This stage is a lot like the unstructured or qualitative interviews we mentioned earlier. The idea is that you spend some time in the setting you want to study, observing and talking to several people fairly informally to establish the boundaries and see what the main issues are. Your informal chats would be focused by the research problem. Working from the notes you make, you are more likely to design a structured questionnaire later on that asks relevant questions. It is usually a mistake to assume that you already know what questions to ask in a survey without exploratory work. You may be biased by your own views.

Pilot study

On the basis of your exploratory work you should now be in a position to draft some semi-structured questions. This means asking questions on the issues raised in the exploratory stage in a way that will elicit the range of answers you are likely to encounter. At this stage it is probably better to leave the questions fairly open ended or allow room for comments, so that people may talk freely on the topics (see Figure 7.2 as an example). In order to assess the range of issues and possible responses, it is a good idea to include between 20 and 50 people in your pilot study, depending on the breadth and depth of topics to be studied.

Main survey

The results of your pilot study should give you enough information to design a structured questionnaire, i.e. closed questions with fixed choice responses such as those in Figure 7.1 (above). The structuring of questions is covered in a later section.

In a very large survey there might be further drafts of the questionnaire or schedule for checking and refining. Even with thorough preparation at the exploratory and pilot stages, it is inevitable that you get the wording of some questions wrong.

If you decide to go ahead on the first draft of the main survey, it is still worth a 'suck it and see' test. Try the questionnaire out on a few handy people to see if they understand all the questions and how to answer them.

It is at this point that decisions about design, question wording and structuring of answers need to be finalised. The size of sample must be decided. Someone with statistical expertise should also be consulted. You might want to consider computer analysis of your results. All of these matters will be dealt with in the rest of the chapter.

SCENARIO

We have already heard in Chapter 5 that Sister Brown has two main lines of enquiry:

1. The likely effects on community nurse work-loads of 5-day surgical units and day units (a quantitative exercise).
2. She also intends to interview a sample of patients and their carers on their feelings about early discharge (a less structured approach).

From this broad beginning she has developed some working hypotheses:

1. Earlier discharge will increase the work-load of the community nurse.
2. Early discharge patients and their carers will express anxiety about coping at home.

To check the first hypothesis Sister Brown needs to design a form for community nurses to record details of their visits over a certain period. She hopes, as a spin-off to the study, that the form could be refined for use on a regular basis as a quality assurance tool.

She decides that the interviews with patients and carers will be more of a pilot study, involving a sample of early discharge patients, and will therefore be semi-structured. A lot of exploratory work has already been covered in her day-to-day visits. Sister Brown would like to continue the study into a larger survey with a structured questionnaire, when day surgery and 5-day stays are introduced to Ward 4, so that the effects on patients and carers can be properly evaluated.

We shall report on Sister Brown's progress again at the end of the chapter.

DESIGN

There are five main rules about questionnaire design:

1. Ask questions that are easy to understand and answer.
2. Give clear instructions.
3. Adopt a format that facilitates analysis.
4. Allow questions to flow to maintain interest.
5. Consider overall impressions.

Ask questions that are easy to understand and answer

Don't overestimate the ability of the respondent. It has been said that the average reading age of the population is 9 years old, and that the *Sun* newspaper is written with that in mind. Too many questionnaires are written in the language of the middle-class professional. Questions should be short and simple.

Give clear instructions

Spell out exactly how the respondent should answer the questions, even if the survey is conducted by interview. Say, for example, whether more than one answer is possible to a multiple-choice question, whether boxes are to be ticked, numbers circled, etc. Figure 7.1 gives some examples, where one box is to be ticked, because only one answer is thought to be possible. An example of a multiple-choice question is shown in Figure 7.4.

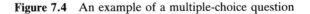

1. How do you get information	Nursing press	☐
on post-registration courses?	Management	☐
(Please tick more than one	School of Nursing	☐
answer if appropriate)	Colleagues	☐
	Other	☐

If 'Other' please specify ....

Figure 7.4 An example of a multiple-choice question

Notice that space is given for comments even in a structured questionnaire so that people can still have some freedom of response.

Make it clear what people should do if they answer 'no' to a question – should they move on to a later question? See the example in Figure 7.5.

1. Have you changed jobs since obtaining the degree?
   (Please tick one box)   Yes   ☐
                                            No   ☐

   If 'Yes' please answer Question 2.
   If 'No' please go to Question 3.

Figure 7.5   An example of a question with instructions for respondents

Another method is to treat the questions like a flow chart and draw arrows to the next appropriate question. You may have noticed that this method is now being used to simplify official forms (see Figure 7.6).

1. Have you changed jobs since obtaining
   the degree?
   (Please tick one box)   YES   NO
                                            ☐   ☐

2. Was the degree a necessary qualification
   for the job?
   (Please tick one box)   YES   NO
                                            ☐   ☐

3. Have you enrolled for any other courses?

Figure 7.6   An example of branching questions

Questionnaires need careful editing for this kind of 'branching' question because respondents can get hopelessly lost among all the different options.

Adopt a format that facilitates analysis

It will be easier and quicker at the analysis stage if all the answers are ranged down the right-hand side of the page as in our examples. Some questionnaires leave an additional column for coding on the right edge of the page, marked 'Office use only' (see Figure 7.1), or 'Please leave blank' or 'Do not write in this column'. We will be dealing with the question of coding later.

Allow questions to flow to maintain interest

Questions should be logically ordered and interesting. The opening questions should grab the respondent's interest, which is why it isn't always sensible to start with personal details such as age, occupation, salary, etc. especially if these include sensitive areas. They may be best left to the end, so that you start straight into the important topics but at a light, non-threatening level at first. Then you can move on to the more weighty matters of interest. The flow of questions can be represented as:

$$Easy \rightarrow Meat \rightarrow Personal\ details$$

In a survey of nurses' views on financial constraints in the NHS, for instance, it would make sense to start the questionnaire with some routine details of how the individual is affected by cuts in their daily work before seeking more political views.

Consider overall impressions

Pay attention to the look of the questionnaire. Is the layout attractive and pleasant to use? What about the length? It should be as short as possible

---

PROFESSIONAL DEVELOPMENT SURVEY

I am a student undertaking a project as part of a course in nursing research methods, and I am interested in the views of qualified nurses in Southshire on the current debate about professional development. I would, therefore, be most grateful if you could complete this short questionnaire and return it as soon as possible to me in the enclosed stamped, addressed envelope. Any details that you give will be anonymous and confidential. I hope to publish the results later in the nursing press. Please let me know if you would like any further details.

Figure 7.7   An example of an introductory paragraph for a questionnaire

otherwise the respondent may become tired and bored or not even bother with the questionnaire. Remember your own experiences with questionnaires.

Be ruthless about which questions you include. Resist the temptation to ask everything connected with the topic that might be interesting, and 'weed out' questions in the final stages. Remember also the amount of data you are generating. If you ask 100 people 20 questions then you will have 2000 bits of data to handle!

Give some introduction to the questionnaire and the topic. You may include this as an introductory paragraph on the questionnaire itself (Figure 7.7) or include a covering letter (Figure 7.8).

Dept of Nursing,
Hightown College,
Southshire

(date)

Dear Colleague,

We are a group of students undertaking a project as part of a course in nursing research methods.

We would like to find out what contribution a part-time nursing degree makes towards professional development. To discover this, we thought it appropriate to canvas a sample of degree graduates throughout the country to find out their career patterns.

A questionnaire is enclosed. When completed, we would be grateful if it could be returned to us in the stamped, addressed envelope. Any details that you give will be anonymous and confidential.

Results of the survey will be published at a later date in the nursing press, or a report will be available from us if required.

Thank you for your help.

Yours faithfully,

Course Representative

Figure 7.8 An example of a covering letter for a questionnaire

In either case you need to interest the reader in the topic, stress its relevance or importance, in order to gain their co-operation. Explain therefore *why* you are doing a survey, *what* it is for and *how* you are doing it.

Always maintain a polite tone – e.g. 'Please tick one answer'. Thank the respondent heartily both before doing the questionnaire (in the introduction or letter) and afterwards – e.g. 'Thank you so much for your help'. You might also want to offer details of the results if people are interested – e.g. 'Please tick this box if you would be interested in receiving details of the results of the survey'.

Don't forget to stress confidentiality and anonymity, as our examples show, if that is what you are offering.

QUESTION WORDING

Remember that people do not always behave in the way the say they do. People generally like to please, so they may try very hard to give you the answer they think you want. The trick is to ask questions in such a way that you get as close as possible to the truth.

Here are some *dos* and *don'ts* on the wording of questions in questionnaires:

> Don't use long complex questions.
> Do keep questions clear and simple.

For example:

> 'Do you think student nurses should get more pay?'

is more straightforward than:

> 'There's been a lot of talk in the media about pay awards for different grades, especially student nurses. What do you think?'

> Don't ask double-barrelled questions.
> Do ask one question at a time.

> 'Are you satisfied with the pay offer or do you think there should be further negotiations?'

is actually two questions in one. If someone answers 'yes', which question are they answering? It needs to be translated into two or more questions.

> Don't ask leading questions.
> Do word questions neutrally.

A leading question runs along the lines of:

> 'Do you agree that . . .?', 'Don't you think it would be a good idea if . . .?' or 'Would it be better if . . .?'

It *leads* the respondent to the answer suggested by the question, rather than finding their own view. An example would be:

'Do you believe that it is unethical for nurses to strike?'

A more neutral approach is to simply invite respondents to state their opinions:

'Please state your views on whether nurses should strike',

or provide a range of views as a multiple-choice question.

Don't ask hypothetical questions.
Do make questions concrete and individual.

'If you were the Prime Minister, what would you do about the NHS?'

is too hypothetical and won't provide very useful information.

'Do you have any suggestions for cost-effective changes in your ward?'

might be more realistic.

Don't ask embarrassing questions.
Do be indirect in sensitive areas.

Direct questions about pay, politics and controversial topics such as abortion are likely to produce guarded responses. Much better to present a range of statements to which people can state their agreement or disagreement.

Don't use vague, ambiguous words.
Do be specific.

'How far do you walk each day?'

is preferable to

'How much exercise do you get?'

Don't use jargon or high-brow words.
Do use simple language.

People will understand:

'Do you take aspirin or paracetamol when the pain starts?'

better than:

'Do you need analgesics?'

Don't ask recall questions.
Do give memory guides.

If you ask questions such as:

'How often do you go to the doctor's?'

you will get inaccurate responses. Guides like:

'How many times have you been to the doctor's in the last week/month/6 months, etc.?'

are more reliable.

> Don't ask proxy questions.
> Do question people direct.

Never ask a wife, say, about her husband's health. Ask him direct.

WAYS OF STRUCTURING ANSWERS

When you are structuring answers on a questionnaire there are alternative types to choose from:

- Open questions
- Yes/No
- Multiple-choice, cafeteria or check-list
- Rank ordering
- Graded alternatives
- Combination of check-list and grading
- Attitude scales

Open questions

We have already referred to open and semi-structured questions and given examples in Figures 7.2 and 7.3 above.

Yes/No

Examples of this type can be found in Figures 7.1 and 7.5 above.

Multiple-choice, cafeteria or check-list

This is the type of question we discussed earlier where one or more answer is possible. An example is given in Figure 7.9.

What does the word 'healthy' mean to you?
(Please tick one or more answers)
  a) Living to be very old   ☐
  b) Never having a cold   ☐
  c) Hardly ever going to the doctor   ☐
  d) Eating the right foods   ☐
  e) Exercising regularly   ☐
  f) Feeling happy and well   ☐
  g) Being able to look after yourself   ☐
  h) Other (please specify below)   ☐

  ....

Figure 7.9   A multiple-choice, cafeteria or check-list question

Rank ordering

The rank order question invites respondents to put a list of items in order of preference or, in other words, to grade or score them. For example, see Figure 7.10.

Please indicate the order of importance to you of these things in life. Place a 1 beside the most important, 2 beside the next most important, and so on:

    a) Achievement at work   —
    b) Family relationships   —
    c) Friendships/social life   —
    d) Health   —
    e) Money   —
    f) Religion   —
    g) Other (please specify below)   —

....

Figure 7.10 An example of a rank-ordering question

A variation on this approach in an interview is to provide the respondents with cards, one for each category, to sort into order of importance.

Graded alternatives

Some examples of this are shown in Figure 7.11.

1. Are you encouraged to apply for study days?
   (Please tick one box)

                 Always   ☐
                 Sometimes   ☐
                 Never   ☐

2. In general, how healthy do you consider yourself?
   (Please tick one box)

                 Very healthy   ☐
                 Fairly healthy   ☐
                 Fairly unhealthy ☐
                 Very unhealthy   ☐

Figure 7.11 Examples of graded alternatives questions

Combination of check-list and grading

The example for this is shown in Figure 7.12. In the example some questions are stated as negatives so that respondents have to consider each one. The tendency when all statements are positive is to tick automatically down the 'agree' columns.

**Please tick one box for each
of the following statements:**

Professional development . . .	Strongly agree	Agree	Disagree	Strongly disagree
a) Keeps you up to date	☐	☐	☐	☐
b) Is not for promotion	☐	☐	☐	☐
c) Is not directly relevant to patient care	☐	☐	☐	☐
d) Helps with teaching students	☐	☐	☐	☐

Figure 7.12 An example of a combined check-list and grading question

Attitude scales

The best known of this type are the Thurstone, Likert and Guttman Scales, and the Semantic Differential technique. They are similar to the graded alternative question type, but more technical. They need to be carefully constructed and tested to be statistically viable. If you are seriously considering this kind of question, we suggest that you refer to one of the guides to survey methods, such as Moser and Kalton (1971), quoted at the end of the chapter. The Repertory Grid is another method, along similar lines, that you may encounter and want to find out more about (Oppenheim, 1966).

On the whole it is best to aim for a balance of answer types including one or two open questions. This gives respondents an interesting variety – it can be very boring to answer a whole series of yes/no or multiple-choice questions. Open questions allow the respondents space for comments and expression of their feelings. In an interview, the interviewer can probe and prompt on open questions. The resulting qualitative data are usually very rich and lend support and substance to quantitative results.

With closed questions the general rule is that categories should be mutually exclusive, exhaustive and not overlapping. A common mistake is to overlap categories such as age bands, as shown in Figure 7.13.

What is your age? **(Tick one box)**	Under 20	☐
	20–25	☐
	25–30	☐
	Over 30	☐

Figure 7.13   An example of a question with overlapping categories – 1

With this banding a person of 20, 25 or 30 could actually tick two boxes.

Similar problems arise over definitions of terms, such as the case in Figure 7.14 where divorced, separated and widowed people would also be single status, and could be a single parent as well, so that an individual might tick three boxes!

What is your marital status? **(Tick one box)**	Married	☐
	Single	☐
	Divorced	☐
	Separated	☐
	Widowed	☐
	Single parent	☐

Figure 7.14   An example of a question with overlapping categories – 2

Exercise

Test your understanding of the rules of question wording and structure by criticising the 'bad' questionnaire in Figure 7.15. How many deliberate mistakes can you find? A good test of any questionnaire, which you might like to try, is to answer the questions yourself, seeing how far you can misinterpret them.

SURVEY OF PATIENTS' VISITORS

1.	How old are you?		—
2.	What is the patient in hospital for?	Minor surgery	☐
		Major surgery	☐
3.	Are you the patient's . . .	Spouse?	☐
		Son/daughter?	☐
		Brother/sister?	☐
4.	Do you think visiting time is organised properly?	Yes	☐
		No	☐
5.	How do you travel to the hospital?	Walk	☐
		Public transport	☐
		By car	☐
6.	Do you agree that sister should speak to all visitors?	Yes	☐
		No	☐
7.	Are you married with children? (Please state how many)		—
8.	Which social class do you belong to?:	Working class	☐
		Middle class	☐
		Upper class	☐

Figure 7.15 An example of a 'bad' questionnaire for exercise

Discussion

Question 1
A startling start to the questionnaire. This type of question is best asked at the end, and in a more indirect way – i.e. 'Which of these age bands applies to you?'

Question 2
Not only is the question asking for information by proxy, it is assuming that the respondent has knowledge of hospital jargon like 'minor' and 'major' surgery.

Question 3
There are no answer categories other than close relatives and no space for others to be added.

Question 4
A vague, unspecified question that is difficult to answer, especially with a yes or no answer. The question needs to be more specific and a range of answers offered, with instructions as to whether one or more answer are possible.

Question 5
The answer categories here overlap. They don't allow for the fact that someone might travel to the hospital by more than one of these methods – e.g. part of the way by bus, part on foot.

Question 6
It sounds as if this is what the survey is all about and the researcher wants to prove a point. A very leading question. Again, with a yes/no response, no room is left for degrees of opinion.

Question 7
This is a double- (or even triple-) barrelled question. With the lack of guidelines, erratic responses are likely.

Question 8
What an embarrassing question! What would *your* response be? If social class is an important variable, it is better to ask for occupation and work out the class by the Registrar General's classification later.

You may have found lots of other points to criticise. It really is a bad questionnaire, but questions similar to these appear regularly in surveys.

Exercise

This exercise can be conducted individually or in a group. It is designed to help you develop a structured questionnaire or interview schedule through exploratory and pilot stages, as follows:

1. Explore a suitable topic for a survey through discussion and observation in the kind of setting you want to study.
2. Refine the topic area by defining specific hypotheses and key variables.
3. Choose the most important variables for the survey.
4. Draft some 'open-ended' questions on these variables.
5. Address these questions to a number of people and record their responses.
6. Decide how each question is best translated into a 'closed' format for a structured questionnaire.
7. Design the order and layout of the questionnaire.

We will return to the exercise after some discussion of sampling.

It is at the design stage that you need to prepare a sample group, although broad decisions about sampling may already have been made at an earlier stage.

Most surveys are based on a sample because, with the exception of the census, there is not enough time or resources to get information on the total group of interest.

Definitions

Sampling is the process of selecting a portion of the population to represent the entire population. A sample, therefore, is a sub-set of a population selected to participate in a research study. A population is the aggregate of all cases of interest with common characteristic(s).

If you wanted to do a survey on drinking and driving, then you would draw your sample from the national population over the age of 16, whereas the population for a survey of nurses might be restricted to qualified nurses in a certain geographical area only.

A major consideration, therefore, is the degree to which the sample represents the population. In particular you need to beware of bias – the under- or over-representation of certain groups. Otherwise you may have to qualify your findings.

In the example of the drinking and driving survey, if our sample contained more women than men and over half were under 30 years of age, we could only report findings that applied to those groups. We could not claim that they were representative of the adult population as a whole.

Rules

There are certain rules to follow in sampling so that you can be more confident about generalising the results of your sample to the rest of the population.

It is generally better if the sampling is based on probability methods, although these are often seen as more costly because they take longer. Probability methods mean that the sample is randomly selected from the population, rather like selecting names from a hat.

Exercise

Imagine that you are arranging an exchange visit for a British hospital of 500 staff with a French hospital, but there is only one coach with 50 places available. What would be the fairest way of sharing out the places?

Discussion

In your suggestions for a solution to this problem you are likely to have discovered for yourself some of the basic principles of sampling. The four most common ways of sampling are:

1. Simple sampling.
2. Stratified sampling.
3. Cluster sampling.
4. Quota sampling.

Simple sampling

This is where you choose randomly from the total population. In our example of the hospital, 500 names could be put in a hat and 50 taken out, like a raffle or a lottery. This can be rather time consuming and so a more straightforward method is to choose 50 names from a list of all the names, either using a random number table to decide the order of choice or by taking every tenth name (calculated from the fraction of 500 divided by 50), perhaps starting with a randomly chosen number.

Stratified sampling

In our example you might have felt that certain groups needed to be represented on the visit – that doctors, nurses, therapists all needed to be represented for instance. Simple random sampling might leave some of them out. Stratified sampling allows for chosen groups to be in a sample by randomly selecting within strata. To choose the sample for our French visit, therefore, we would first decide on the groups or strata (doctors, nurses, therapists, etc.) and then make a simple random choice within each group. Say we had 5 groups to be represented, we could choose 10 from each group, although the number might depend on the size of each group. If there were twice as many nurses as doctors for instance we might choose 13 nurses and 7 doctors – unless somebody argued that doctors were more important and needed more representatives!

Cluster sampling

Let's extend our exercise a little and imagine that the coach from our hospital is one of several going from all over Britain. The selection of coach loads could have been achieved by cluster sampling, which is a two-stage process of randomly chosen clusters. For example, some national organisation could have been invited by French authorities to arrange for 10 coaches to visit. To be as fair as possible the organisers could have chosen 10 hospitals in simple random fashion from all British hospitals and then instructed each hospital to make a random choice of 50 as we discussed above.

Quota sampling

This kind of sampling is not based on random methods but on the principle of fulfilling certain quotas. It has been developed mainly in the field of market research. You may have had the experience of being approached in the street by a market researcher saying, 'I've been looking for a woman of your age'!

To return to our example, we could have decided in advance how many of each profession we wanted to be represented on the French visit, according to some criteria such as relevance or importance. Say we decided on 10 of each of 5 groups: doctors, nurses, therapists, administrators, health authority members. We could then go to each group and ask for 10 people to be nominated to fill our quota for that group.

In most surveys, a stratified sample is best because it helps to ensure that the sample is representative on key variables, for example, speciality, qualification. The quota method is not so favoured because of the possibility of bias, but it is quicker and cheaper than random choice methods. There are times when one may have to compromise because there is not the freedom to choose a random sample. If, for example, you wanted to survey the views of nurses locally on a particular topic, but could not get access to computerised staff records to work out a random sample, you might estimate a quota sample and approach colleagues with a reasonable balance of age and experience.

Size of sample

There is no hard and fast rule about sample size. A rough rule of thumb is to use as large a sample as possible. Aim for more than a hundred if you want to include different groups, and do quite a lot of statistics with your data. Two to three hundred is a respectable number if you are doing a serious survey. Any more might become unmanageable.

The size of sample will of course depend on the size of the total population and the variety of groups within it that need to be represented. With certain groups it might be feasible to use the whole population – for example, all trained nurses in a hospital or district.

Exercise

Consider the questionnaire from the previous exercise. Decide the most appropriate sample size. Choose an appropriate sampling method from simple, stratified, cluster and quota sampling methods.

INTERVIEW SKILLS

If you are doing your survey via interviews, the necessary social skills would have to be taken into account. Interviews are discussed again in more detail in the chapter on qualitative methods but we would just like to stress here the importance of attending to skills because the interview has to be handled properly as a brief social interaction between strangers. We mentioned earlier the importance of consistency in approach between interviewers. In large surveys interviewers are trained before the survey starts and the matching between interviewer and respondent is carefully considered.

Rate of response can be a problem, especially with postal and self-completion questionnaires. The number of questionnaires returned can obviously vary between 0% and 100%. As we discussed earlier, it is important that the sample is representative of the population and if a large proportion of the sample does not respond, the sample may become biased. Non-responders can differ from responders on key characteristics that influence their ability or time to respond. Men tend to be worse responders than women. The elderly, the rurally based and lower socioeconomic groups seem to find it more difficult to respond.

The accepted 'cut-off' rate for response to surveys is 65%, although the higher the better. Some quite respectable surveys, however, have reported results from lower rates of response.

Strategies

Different strategies have been suggested to overcome the problems of non-response *before* and *after* the survey. More details of these can be found in the references at the end of the chapter.

Before

Careful pilot work and a well-designed questionnaire with a covering letter will go a long way to reducing non-response. A stamped addressed envelope can help, although this adds to the cost of the survey, of course. If you can engage people's interest, they are more likely to respond. Sometimes incentives are used, such as copies of the results or an invitation to a meeting. Market research firms often offer free gifts.

After

Reminders can be effective if firm and timed right. Hoinville and Jowell (1977) suggest that responses can be boosted by 20% (from around 40% to 60%) after a first reminder, 10 days after the initial mailing and a further 10% (up to 80+ %) after a second reminder at around 20 days. Some researchers send another copy of the questionnaire with the second reminder.

Non-responders are sometimes followed up personally with an interview. This is not possible if the questionnaire was anonymous.

The responses to follow-ups can be used as a sample of the non-responders and as a check on any bias in the group of responders. If necessary the results could be weighted to compensate for bias.

In the case of non-response because people refuse, have moved on or are on holiday, you could select a substitute with matching characteristics.

CODING RESULTS

Results from questionnaires that are to be analysed statistically by computer need to be coded into number form ready for 'punching in' or processing by the computer programme. Figure 7.16 shows how responses to our earlier sample questionnaire in Figure 7.1 have been coded in the right-hand column. Alternatively, the codes can be transferred to a 'coding sheet' that eases and speeds up the 'punching in' (see Figure 7.17). There is a box for each digit and space for the results from several questionnaires.

The conventions for converting results to codes are fairly straightforward. In simple 'yes/no' categorisation, 'Yes' is coded as 1 and 'No' as 2. A list of items in a multiple-choice question is numbered from 1 onwards as in our example in Figure 7.16 above. In a multiple-choice question that allows for more than one answer, however, each item on the list needs to be treated as if it was a separate 'yes/no' question and rated 1 or 2 according to whether it has a tick or not. To take the example given in Figure 7.9 under the heading 'Multiple choice, cafeteria and check-list' respondents were invited to tick one or more answers from a list of statements about health. Each statement ticked would be coded 1 as if it was a separate question where the response was 'Yes'. Any statements not ticked would be coded 2, the equivalent of a 'No.'

Missing data are conventionally coded 9.

To guide and interpret coding, you need to write a 'coding frame'. The coding frame for our example in Figures 7.16 and 7.17 would read something like Figure 7.18 (p. 103).

You might find you want more guidelines on coding so some useful references are given at the end of the chapter (Oppenheim, 1966; Moser and Kalton, 1971; Hoinville and Jowell, 1977).

Any additional comments on a questionnaire, such as those made under 'Please specify' in our examples, can be analysed qualitatively (see Chapter 8 for discussion) or counted using a form of 'content analysis' (see Chapter 5) to be included on the coding sheet. This involves listing and tallying the most frequent responses to each question and combining them into categories so that the question can be treated as a multiple-choice type. The number of categories should ideally be less than 9, so that 9 can be used as the code for missing data. Figure 7.19 (p. 104) gives an example of the process for the open question 'Name one personal health issue that worries you', and the resulting codes in Figure 7.20 (p. 105).

WHERE ARE YOU NOW?

Office use

If you are a part-time nursing degree graduate we would be grateful if you could answer the following questions:

1. In which area was your career *before* the degree?
   (Please tick one box)

Clinical/Community	☑	1
Education	☐	
Management	☐	
Other	☐	

   (if 'Other' please specify)

   ....

2. In which area was your career *during* the degree?
   (Please tick one box)

Clinical/Community	☐	2
Education	☑	
Management	☐	
Other	☐	

   (if 'Other' please specify)

   ....

3. In which area was your career *after* the degree?
   (Please tick one box)

Clinical/Community	☐	2
Education	☑	
Management	☐	
Other	☐	

   (if 'Other' please specify)

   ....

4. Are you . . .
   (Please tick one box)

Female?	☑	1
Male?	☐	

5. Do you have any other comments?
   (Please write overleaf)

   2

MANY THANKS FOR YOUR HELP

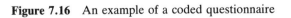

Figure 7.16   An example of a coded questionnaire

'WHERE ARE YOU NOW?' SURVEY

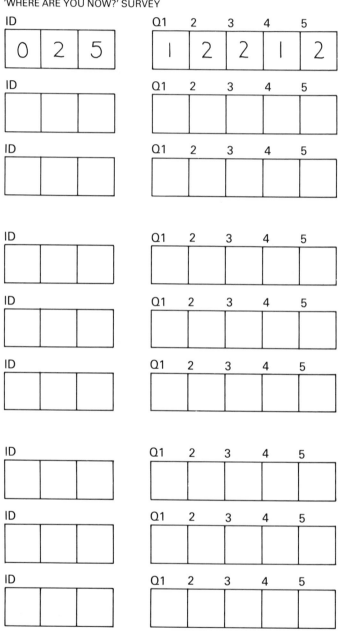

Figure 7.17 An example of a coding sheet

```
WHERE ARE YOU NOW? SURVEY

Coding Frame
ID    001–150
Q1.   1 = Clinical/Community
      2 = Education
      3 = Management
      4 = Other
Q2.   (as for Q1)
Q3.   (as for Q1)
Q4.   1 = Female
      2 = Male
Q5.   1 = Comments made
      2 = No comments
```

Figure 7.18   An example of a coding frame

Once the data have been processed, they are ready for analysis by one of the many statistical packages available for small and large computers. We do strongly recommend anybody who is interested in using computers to analyse their data to seek advice at an early stage on the design and coding of the questionnaire and on the most suitable computer package for analysis.

We will resume our discussion of data analysis in Chapter 10.

SCENARIO

Remember that Sister Brown was working on two hypotheses in her survey of the effect of early discharge on patients and carers? These were:

1.   Earlier discharge will increase the work-load of the community nurse.
2.   Early discharge patients and their carers will express anxiety about coping at home.

Visiting times

The forms that Sister Brown designed to record visiting times are shown in Figures 7.21 and 7.22 (pp. 106 and 107). She has chosen to collect data over a 2-month period for all surgical patients in the hospital. She is aiming for a return on around 90 patients. To achieve this she has had to obtain the co-operation of a wide circle of colleagues in the hospital and in the community. The clinical nurse managers in the community have agreed to collect the records from community nurses. A note explaining the purpose of the study has been circulated to all the community nurses beforehand.

Q1. Name one personal health issue that worries you

		TOTAL
Stroke	|	1
Infectious diseases	|	1
Rheumatism	||	2
Smoking	┼┼┼┼ ┼┼┼┼	10
Eczema	|	1
Heart disease	┼┼┼┼ ┼┼┼┼ |	11
AIDS	┼┼┼┼ ┼┼┼┼ ┼┼┼┼ ┼┼┼┼ ||||	24
Being overweight	┼┼┼┼ |	6
Cancer	┼┼┼┼ ┼┼┼┼ ┼┼┼┼ ┼┼┼┼ ┼┼┼┼ ┼┼┼┼ ┼┼┼┼||	37
Arthritis	┼┼┼┼ ┼┼┼┼ |	11
Diabetes	|||	3
Kidneys	||	2
Stress	┼┼┼┼ |||	8
Alcohol	|	1
Not eating right food	||	2
Allergies	||||	4
Asthma	||	3
Becoming disabled	||	2
Sinus	|	1
Blood pressure	|	1
Lack of exercise	|	1
Back problems	┼┼┼┼	5
Leukaemia	|	1
Breast cancer	|	1
Ageing	|||	3
Overdoing exercise	|	1
Thyroid problems	|	1
Depression	|	1

Figure 7.19 An example of 'content analysis' of responses to open question

```
┌─────────────────────────────┐
│                             │
│  Coding frame               │
│                             │
│  1 = Cancer                 │
│  2 = AIDS                   │
│  3 = Heart disease          │
│  4 = Smoking                │
│  5 = Stress                 │
│  6 = Weight                 │
│  7 = Arthritis              │
│  8 = Other                  │
│                             │
└─────────────────────────────┘
```

Figure 7.20   A coding frame for the open question in Figure 7.19

As a check on the community data, Sister Jones has offered to provide data on the number of patients referred from different surgical areas for community nurse support. The data can be gathered from the referral forms completed by the hospital liaison sisters. Sister Jones has asked them to make duplicates of the forms over the 2-month period.

Some of the data collected by the forms will be used for exercises in Chapter 10 on data analysis.

Patients and carers

The subjects for semi-structured interviews are selected from the community nurse records. Sister Brown plans to approach around 20 patients who have been discharged after fewer than 5 days. We said earlier that Sister Brown will need the consent of the ethical committee. She will also need the consent of individual patients and their respective carers. The consent form she has drafted is shown in Figure 7.23 (p. 108).

In designing the interview schedule she must bear in mind that community nurses already have a tight time schedule – that is the theme of her study. She, therefore, keeps the schedules short and to the point. These are reproduced in Figures 7.24 and 7.25 (pp. 109 and 110). Note that she has produced one schedule for patients and one for carers because she realises she cannot gauge the feelings of the carer by asking the patient, and vice versa.

With the results of her interviews, Sister Brown would be able to construct a structured questionnaire, with mainly closed questions, for use with a much larger sample. This could be used with patients from her own ward to evaluate the proposed changes. In this case the sample would be aggregated over time with successive patients.

Please complete all sections

Ward/hospital discharged from: _____

Date of discharge: _____

Date of first visit: _____

Date of final visit: _____

Operation: _____

Operation date: _____

Liaison form received: yes/no (delete as appropriate)

If patient treated in treatment room/general practitioner surgery by district nurse, use initials T/R in appropriate timings box.

If treatment given at general practitioner surgery by practice nurse, please indicate under comments.

Hospital assessment of treatment needs on referral:

District nurse assessment of needs:

Comments:

Figure 7.21 A form for recording details of community nurse visits – 1

Patient's name _____   General practitioner _____

Month	1		2		3		4		5		6		7		8		9		10		11		12		13		14		15		16	
Minutes	a.m.	p.m.	a.m.	p.m.	a.m.	p.m.	a.m.	p.m.	a.m.	p.m.	a.m.	p.m.	a.m.	p.m.	a.m.	p.m.	a.m.	p.m.	a.m.	p.m.	a.m.	p.m.	a.m.	p.m.	a.m.	p.m.	a.m.	p.m.	a.m.	p.m.	a.m.	p.m.
Less than 15																																
Up to 30																																
Up to 50																																
Up to 60																																
60+																																

Month	17		18		19		20		21		22		23		24		25		26		27		28		29		30		31	
Minutes	a.m.	p.m.	a.m.	p.m.	a.m.	p.m.	a.m.	p.m.	a.m.	p.m.	a.m.	p.m.	a.m.	p.m.	a.m.	p.m.	a.m.	p.m.	a.m.	p.m.	a.m.	p.m.	a.m.	p.m.	a.m.	p.m.	a.m.	p.m.	a.m.	p.m.
Less than 15																														
Up to 30																														
Up to 50																														
Up to 60																														
60+																														

Figure 7.22   A form for recording details of community nurse visits – 2

SOUTHSHIRE HEALTH AUTHORITY

COMMUNITY SURVEY: COPING AT HOME AFTER SURGERY

Informed Consent Form

As community nurses, we are interested to find out how surgery patients and their carers cope at home after a short stay in hospital, and the kind of support they need.

We would, therefore, like to interview some patients and their main carers (if appropriate). Each interview would be conducted by a community nurse, Sister Brown, and would last no more than half an hour. All information will be treated confidentially both during and after the study. Sister Brown would be happy to discuss any questions you might have (Telephone 54321).

If you consent to take part in the study, we would be grateful if you could complete the tear-off slip below and give it to your local community nurse.

....

COMMUNITY SURVEY: COPING AT HOME AFTER SURGERY

This is to certify that .... (print name) CAN/CANNOT (please delete as appropriate) participate in the above-named study, and that I DO/DO NOT (please delete) give permission for information given in an interview to be recorded in written form. I understand that all material will be treated as highly confidential by the researcher. I have been given the opportunity to ask any questions, and know that I am free to withdraw my consent at any time.

Signed ....

Date ....

Figure 7.23 An example of a consent form

COMMUNITY SURVEY: COPING AT HOME AFTER SURGERY

Patient Interview Schedule

1. How long were you in hospital?

2. Did you feel ready to come home?

3. Were you given details about your condition (if so, by whom)?

4. Do you feel you were given enough information?

5. Do you have a carer at home (if so, details of who)?

6. Do you have any particular problems coping at home
   (domestic arrangements, etc.)?

7. How will you manage?

8. Do you have any other worries?

9. Is there anything you think you need?

THANKS FOR YOUR HELP

Figure 7.24   Community survey interview schedule – 1

COMMUNITY SURVEY: COPING AT HOME AFTER SURGERY

Carer Interview Schedule

1. What is your relationship to the patient?

2. Did you feel ready to look after the patient at home?

3. Were you given details about the patient's condition (if so, by whom)?

4. Do you feel you were given enough information?

5. How much support do you need to give to the patient?

6. Do you have any particular problems coping at home (domestic arrangements, etc.)?

7. How will you manage?

8. Do you have any other worries?

9. Is there anything you think you need?

THANKS FOR YOUR HELP

Figure 7.25   Community survey interview schedule – 2

BIBLIOGRAPHY

Clark J M and Hockey L (1979) *Research for Nursing: A Guide for the Enquiring Nurse.* London: H M and M Publishers.

Clark J M and Hockey L (1988) *Further Research for Nursing: A New Guide for the Enquiring Nurse.* London: Scutari Press.

Cormack D F S (1984) *The Research Process in Nursing,* chs 9 and 11. Oxford: Blackwell.

Hoinville G and Jowell R (1977) *Survey Research Practice.* London: Heinemann.

Moser J A and Kalton G (1971) *Survey Methods in Social Investigations.* London: Heinemann.

Oppenheim A N (1966) *Questionnaire Design and Attitude Measurement.* London: Heinemann.

Polit D and Hungler B (1983) *Nursing Research: Principles and Methods,* chs 7, 9 and 11. Philadelphia: J B Lippincott.

Treece E W and Treece J W (1977) *Elements of Research in Nursing.* New York: C V Mosby.

Wilson-Barnett J (ed.) (1983) *Nursing Research: Ten Studies in Patient Care.* Chichester: John Wiley and Sons.

8

Qualitative Techniques

Student Nurse Green decides that, as part of the ward's research, it would be useful to find out what kinds of thing patients worry about on going home after having had an operation. That would help the ward staff in preparing patients for discharge if the length of stay were to be reduced. However, she does not really have very much time to devote to the research and if she wants to interview patients, she will have to get ethical approval first, which could take time. On the other hand, is it possible to carry out research at the same time as working on the ward?

The purpose of this chapter is to discuss the advantages and disadvantages of different qualitative techniques, to explore some of the issues in qualitative research and to describe some of the ways of analysing this type of data.

If you look back at Chapter 5 on research design, you will see that we talked there of the spectrum of nursing, theory development and qualitative and quantitative methods. You will remember that the key issue in research design was the place of the study in relation to these concepts.

So we come back to the point that there are research situations in which qualitative techniques will be the most appropriate and others where they will not.

Qualitative methods are generally regarded as being less 'scientific', less concerned with establishing causality, descriptive rather than explanatory, exploratory rather than testing. Qualitative methods work from the particular to the general (inductive logic) whereas quantitative methods, with their hypothesis testing and high dependence on statistical significance of findings, work from the general to the particular (deductive logic).

Having described qualitative methods as less scientific, the point needs to be made that this does not mean that you can afford to be less rigorous in conducting qualitative research. All the problems concerned with ensuring validity, reliability and reactivity are just as applicable. In fact, in some ways these issues are even more important, because they are not 'built in' by nature of the research design, so you have to take more trouble to see that these factors are taken into account.

Although qualitative research is thought of as being exploratory in nature, many research projects use entirely qualitative methods, particularly in the social sciences. Others use qualitative methods followed by quantitative methods to test out some of the relationships indicated in the first phase. You could say that in the qualitative/quantitative debate it is a question of 'horses for courses'.

Field and Morse (1985) give helpful definitions of the different approaches at the qualitative end of the research methods continuum. All the approaches share the attempt to understand society from the perspective of the participants themselves but differ in their depth of analysis.

There are two main methods of collecting qualitative data; interview and observation. In addition, some of the methods listed in Chapter 5 can be used to collect qualitative data. Documents such as diaries and letters, for instance, or the game simulation technique, could be used in this way.

INTERVIEWS

Just as qualitative and quantitative methods were discussed earlier as being at either end of a continuum, so interviews range from structured to unstructured. Figure 8.1 explains how this affects the data collected.

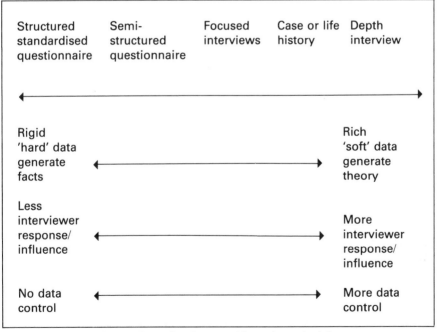

Figure 8.1   Continuum of interview schedule

Setting up the interviews needs to be carefully planned. When you first contact the people to be interviewed (called respondents), a convenient and suitable time and place for the next meeting must be agreed. This may only be a preliminary visit so you can explain what is required and what is expected of the respondent and to gain consent. More than one interview may be necessary with each respondent, and if you feel this is likely, you should be honest and say so. The respondents should, when consent is sought, be clearly told that they may withdraw from the study at any time. It is a good idea to leave a letter explaining as simply as possible the purpose of the study and the name and telephone number of whom to contact if they have any queries or worries. The letter should repeat that respondents are under no obligation to participate and that they may withdraw from the study at any time. If children or other vulnerable groups are involved, permission must be sought from a responsible person. The ethical implications of research with vulnerable groups is explored in Chapter 9.

Structured, standardised questionnaire

In this type of interview every respondent is asked exactly the same set of questions with exactly the same wording and in the same order.

The rationale for this is that by providing the same stimulus to each person interviewed, the responses will be comparable. The person conducting the interviews will have less influence on the answers – as long as they stick to the questionnaire.

There are several problems with this type of interview:

1. Not all of the people being interviewed will interpret the wording in the same way. This can be partly overcome by a good pilot study of the questionnaire before the main study commences. Wording should be clear and unambiguous and there should be no double-barrelled questions, or complex sentences.
2. By providing a very rigid set of questions, respondents may be forced into a very rigid set of answers.
3. Such an interview is very artificial. The questions being asked may not provide the opportunity for the respondent to say how he or she really feels about the issue being discussed.

Interviews that use standardised, structured questionnaires are most suitable for obtaining 'facts' rather than 'feelings'.

Thus they can be seen as more to the quantitative end of the methodology spectrum and more akin to a survey approach, but they do have their place in qualitative research. Designing structured questionnaires is a skilled task. Chapter 7 covers various survey methods more fully and explains how to construct such research tools.

Semi-structured questionnaire

In this type of interview you are able to use more complex questions and to 'probe' for more information. What does the word 'engineer' mean for example in response to a question on occupation? It could mean telephone engineer, mechanical engineer or nuclear engineer. Probing enables you to clarify answers to questions.

Semi-structured questionnaires all ask the same questions, but are not so rigid. You can rephrase the question if the respondent does not understand it or clarify something that was confusing. Interviews that use questionnaires can provide information, such as the number of times someone has been in hospital or the last time they visited the doctor, but they cannot provide really perceptive data on how people felt about the experience.

Focused interview

A focused, or guided, interview is rather different. For this, you start out with a list of issues about the particular topic that you wish to cover, but the interview is much more like a conversation. In this way the topics can be discussed as they arise and in the respondent's own words, rather than in the order and format prescribed on a questionnaire. A much wider range of data can be collected in this way, with much more depth. The respondents may raise issues about a topic that you had not thought of or considered unimportant or unlikely. Data collected like this are said to be much 'richer'.

Because of their nature, focused interviews can become rather painful or uncomfortable for respondent and interviewer. You need to be quite skilled at behaving in a way that is non-directive and non-judgmental, but supportive.

Whereas a structured questionnaire has all the information recorded in coded form on the questionnaire itself, this is only partly true of semi-structured questionnaires and not at all for focused interviews.

Tape-recorders are invaluable here and, provided they are sensitively introduced and used, are increasingly well accepted. By using a tape-recorder, you are freed from the task of writing copious notes, and can concentrate on the respondent, watching for non-verbal as well as verbal cues in following up answers.

The tape-recorder should not be placed in too conspicuous a position and small microphones may be helpful. If respondents are embarrassed or hesitant over being recorded, more general conversation at the start of the interview can usually overcome this. Once a more relaxed atmosphere is established the tape-recorder will generally be forgotten and the interview proper can proceed.

Focused interviews are used to explore attitudes or beliefs about some-thing. Although they can form the major part of a research design, focused interviews are also useful for pilot studies as a preliminary stage in the construction of more formal questionnaires. By eliciting the perceptions and viewpoint of a small sample of the research subjects, the researcher is guided on the questions and perhaps wording of a subsequent questionnaire to be administered to the main research sample.

Whether the interview is the administration of a structured questionnaire or a focused interview, you must keep certain things in mind.

First, even when the interview is conducted informally, it is not a normal social interaction. You and your respondents are probably strangers to each other and the encounter will be transitory in nature. This can be an advantage in that respondents may be more frank with someone they never expect to meet again. Differences in class, age and sex between the respondent and yourself may affect the rapport that this technique requires. Also, the two of you are not on an equal footing in that the respondent is the novice and you are the expert in the situation.

Second, it may be difficult to keep the respondent to the point! Although some anecdotal or unrelated matter may be unavoidable, you need to stay in control of the interview. At the same time, avoid giving – even when asked – advice and opinions or imposing your own perspective on the material the respondent is presenting.

Third, interviews can take quite a long time. It is important to minimise distractions or interruptions from others not directly concerned, other members of the respondent's family for instance. Bear this in mind when arranging the time and place of the interview.

There are two other types of interviews that are worth knowing about, but that are not really suitable for the inexperienced or first-time researcher.

Case or life histories

A case or life history is similar to a focused interview in that it allows respondents to give their own account in their own words. However, case or life histories are more autobiographical and will have much wider ranging subject matter. Case histories can be of events, organisations or specific settings, as well as of individuals. Thus a case history could be of one family's experience with a disabled child over a period of several years. Davis' study 'Passage through crisis' was conducted in this way (Davis, 1963). The case history could be concerned with the establishment, organisation and achievements of a new health clinic. Interviews are obviously on-going, being conducted over a long period of time, and may involve interviews with more than one person.

This kind of study obviously requires a great deal of commitment on the part of a researcher and indeed more than one researcher is often involved in this type of work.

Depth interview

In a depth interview there is more interaction between participants. This may develop almost to the point of counselling with the researcher reflecting and clarifying what the respondent says. The point of this is to get at 'hidden' or 'difficult' data, particularly with deviant or unusual subjects, and can, therefore, be very difficult to conduct. Depth interviews can be useful as a prelude to formulating the interview schedule for focused interviews.

OBSERVATION

Observation can be classified into two types:

Observing specific events

In this type of observation you would have decided beforehand exactly what you are looking for.

This is likely to be some kind of 'count' of things, such as the number of times the ward sister answers the telephone in a given period or how often patients in a day hospital initiate conversation with a nurse.

Observing situations

You may want to observe a setting in order to understand what is happening. This may be:

1. To find the reason for particular events.
2. To test a theory or hypothesis around which the research is designed.
3. To generate theory.

There are two points to make here. First, both types of observation may be the only method of data collection, but they are more likely to be used in conjunction with other methods. For example, observation to understand the organisation of a ward may bring to light the fact that the ward sister spends a lot of time on the telephone, in which case observation that specifically counted and timed this activity could follow. Conversely, if observation started by concentrating on this 'telephone-time', the next stage could be to see how this affects the rest of the ward staff.

Second, you have to decide on the role you intend to adopt – in other words how will you explain your presence and how much will you take part in what is going on? Figure 8.2 shows the range of involvement in research settings. Each situation has its advantages and disadvantages and you must decide which is the most appropriate for your particular study.

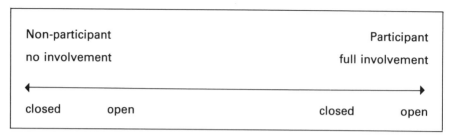

Figure 8.2   Range of observer roles

Non-participant

As a non-participant you will take on no role or task other than that of observer.

This relates not only to activities – such as helping with bed-making! – but also, as far as possible, to not engaging in anything that changes or distorts the setting, which may include conversation with those being observed. The objective is to become a 'fly on the wall'.

Non-participant observation may be 'open' or 'closed'. As this implies, open observation is when the subjects know they are being observed, closed observation is when they do not – or do not know the true purpose.

The question you may be asking about non-participant observation is 'don't people change their behaviour once they know you are watching?' This is called the Hawthorne effect, after a famous series of studies carried out in the USA. In fact, people usually become accustomed to observation quite quickly. In any case, it is difficult to sustain a different pattern of behaviour over a long period of time and in a consistent fashion. Open observation does have the advantage that the appearance of the researcher at meetings and in various locations is explained and people will not be surprised if you ask questions or look at records.

Closed non-participant observation is more difficult for several reasons. If the closed context has been achieved by giving a different reason than the true one or subjects are unaware that they are being observed, then clearly ethical issues arise. In practical terms, how can subjects be observed without their knowledge? Public places such as waiting areas or canteens do not present too much of a problem as you can become one of the crowd, though considerable skill and discretion over note-taking will be necessary. But what about a clinical area? In some research one-way mirrors or hidden cameras have been used. Once again, the ethical considerations are major and additionally such techniques may not allow adequate data collection, as the most important and informative events may occur just out of sight or earshot.

Participant observation

Some research settings and questions can best be investigated when the researcher takes part in the setting itself. Thus if the research is about what topics of conversation are initiated by patients, you could become one of the ward team.

Obviously you need to negotiate a role in the setting prior to or immediately upon starting the data collection. What that role is will depend on whether the observation is open or closed, as in non-participant observation, meaning whether the subjects know what or if research is being carried out. Open participation may have an effect on the behaviour of others, but you will have more understanding of what form this takes. However, do not lose sight of the observer role by remaining objective and impartial and not taking any action that will affect the behaviour or structure of the setting. On the other hand, the advantages of open, non-participant observation are enhanced. Others in the setting will tend to forget your 'other' role after a while and accept your presence and questions.

Closed participant observation may be the only method possible if the research setting is somewhat contentious, for instance with drug addicts or other groups who might resent being the subject of investigation. Apart from the ethical problems here, the role the researcher adopts has to be very carefully chosen and scrupulously maintained. Again, you must remain objective and not allow your assumed role to influence or disturb the behaviour of others.

Clearly, observation studies require tact, sensitivity and a great deal of delicacy if they are to be successful.

One-way mirrors

Observations can be carried out by the use of one-way mirrors, but clearly there are considerable ethical problems with this. If you are observing a situation in which respondents are unaware of this, you are guilty of exploiting them and invading their privacy. On the other hand, if they are aware that you are observing, how much will their behaviour change?

RECORDING THE DATA

Recording the observation as completely as possible is very important. If the observation is of a structured nature, you will need to have an observation schedule prepared. For example, if you were observing the frequency and content of telephone calls on a ward and who answered them, the possible options could be set out in such a way that you could just tick the appropriate boxes for each call observed. Just what these options were would have been developed from notes of earlier unstructured observations in the setting. Both notes and prestructured recording schedules should be made on the spot when this is feasible or as soon after events occur as possible. If you are working in a closed context, this may mean frequent trips to the toilet or repeated visits to a cupboard!

How and what to record

The first stage in observing a situation will be largely unstructured. The purpose will be to get the 'feel', notice patterns or routines of behaviour. This stage may provide data to define classification or degree or start ideas. The second stage will be more structured. Confirmation and checking of concepts identified in the first stage takes place or the objective and focus of the observation becomes narrowed. Notes will vary, according to the stage and purpose of the observation. However you should keep three sets of notes:

Field notes

These are the record of the observation itself and should be made at the time or very soon after leaving the setting. The example below is of a nurse–patient interaction:

> *Nurse (approaching bed)* 'Time to get up Mrs Jones.'
> *Mrs Jones (eyes shut)* 'I don't feel well enough.'
> *Nurse (draws screens)* 'I'm sure you'll feel better out of bed.'
> *Nurse takes clothes out of locker.* Mrs Jones struggles to sit up, then falls back onto pillow. Nurse assists Mrs Jones to sit up. Nurse begins to help Mrs Jones out of nightdress. Neither speaks.

Field notes should be in 'native language' – that is as used by participants and verbatim if possible. If the observation is of action not speech then be as specific as possible.

Personal field work journal

A journal is used to record significant events, such as meetings attended or changes to the organisation or staffing of the setting.

Ideas on analysis and interpretation

As the research proceeds, you may get some clues about how to analyse the data. Similarities (or differences) may suggest concepts, categories or explanations worth pursuing. For instance, the observation recorded in the example could lead to two different concepts:

1. Nurse strategies to obtain patient compliance.
2. Token resistance by patient to demonstrate independence.

Write such ideas down or you may forget them.

Exercises

1. Find a setting you think would be interesting to observe, not

necessarily to do with nursing. Experience has shown that places like launderettes, bus-stations, amusement arcades and pubs can provide rich and amusing data, and this is a useful but lighthearted way to start learning how to observe. When deciding on a setting, use your imagination! Spend about 2 hours on the observation, making notes of what you observe. Try to make some sense of what is going on and see if you can determine any pattern to what you notice. How many people are there? What kinds of people? What are they doing? Why are they behaving like that?

Once you have completed your observation session, write it up as you would if you were going to spend 5 minutes or so telling your colleagues at work about it. If you can find a captive audience, so much the better!

2. Get together with two or three of your friends or colleagues. Decide on a setting for undertaking non-participant observation. A public setting like a waiting area is best, but make sure that you have permission from the relevant staff beforehand. Observe the setting for about an hour, recording any gestures, talk or movement that occur. At this stage, just basic observational data are recorded with as little inference as possible. Do not confer with each other until the end of the observation period, then compare notes and try to suggest some pattern, explanation or theory for the events you have observed.

If this is a class activity, the material collected is analysed, looking for the sociological features of the situation, the categories and concepts that are suggested, the 'roles' of participants, and the 'rules' governing interaction, including departures from these 'rules'. The data will be used to support the theoretical ideas.

3. This exercise is larger in scale and scope. The object is to report, interpret and analyse a social event from the perspective of the people involved, using unstructured observation or interview methods. Select a social event in your work setting in which you already share some of the cultural norms (i.e. you know how people behave and what goes on) and to which you have access. For instance, you might look at the ways in which fellow nurses 'negotiate' their relationships with other professionals.

Decide on a setting for the observation. You will need to negotiate your own access and obtain permission, and remember that if clients or patients are involved, ethical approval will be necessary. Observation is carried out over a period of several days or weeks depending on the time available. Data should be analysed sequentially with data collection, so that the field of inquiry is increasingly narrowed and focused, and theoretical concepts are checked out as they emerge from analysis.

Write a report of at least one thousand words that covers:

1. A brief introduction to the setting.

2. Justification of the method used.
3. How the exercise was conducted.
4. A description of the social event, including passages of dialogue where appropriate.
5. Interpretation and discussion of results, grounded theoretically in the data and in the light of other existing theories.
6. An evaluation of methods and findings of the exercise.

ANALYSING QUALITATIVE DATA

As with deciding on what method to use to study a particular research question, the analysis undertaken will depend on the purpose of the research.

Interviews

No matter what kinds of interview have been conducted, considerable work is necessary before the analysis proper can begin. Structured and semi-structured questionnaires must be scrutinised and coded. Responses to open-ended questions will have to be classified prior to coding. Depending on the size of the sample, the data can be put on to computer for analysis or analysed manually. The researcher is looking for relationships between the variables of the study. For instance, does the age of a diabetic patient correlate with diet compliance? (The variables here are 'age' and 'diet compliance'.) Statistical techniques will be required to establish the validity of such relationships. The analysis of questionnaires is explained more fully. in Chapter 10.

Interviews that have been tape-recorded must be typed up to form a transcript. As a rule of thumb, transcribing will take three times as long as the original interview. Interviews not tape-recorded must be checked for clarity and probably also transcribed to allow analysis. Always make three copies of a transcript, then if disaster strikes you will not lose all your data. Put the original tapes or notes away in a safe place – do not use them as working documents for the analysis.

Observation notes

As with interview data, preparation is required before analysis is started. Make sure your notes are in the right sequence, and if the writing is not clear type the notes into a transcript, making three copies. You may wish to make separate copies of conversations you have recorded, so that you can make a preliminary analysis of both conversation and events before seeing how one reinforces or is different from the other. Have you recorded the outcome of any meetings you attended or followed up any loose ends that

remained when you left the research setting? If you were using a prestructured recording schedule, look all the sheets over and discard any that are
'spoiled' or plainly inaccurate. If any groupings are required, such as into
separate weeks of observation, sort the recording sheets out as necessary.

Analysis

The next step is to read the transcripts through at least twice. Does anything
significant strike you? Are the same phrases, actions or attitudes recurring?
If so, can you classify them – do some of the responses or events seem to
express certain concepts, guilt or frustration, for example? Consult your
field work journal and your 'ideas' notes. Is there anything there to give you
a lead?

How you proceed from here is a matter of personal choice. Some
researchers use highlighter pens to mark categories and concepts on the
portions of transcript. Thus all sections that refer to 'guilt' would be
highlighted in red, 'frustration' in blue and so on. The transcript can be
scrutinised for other concepts or sub-categories of the existing ones. Always
keep one transcript unmarked.

Another method is to cut out the parts of a transcript referring to a
particular concept, such as 'fear', stick each one onto a blank sheet of paper,
then file according to classification. If some sections can be classified in more
than one way, the second copy of the transcript comes into service.

Yet another way is to copy the relevant parts of the transcript onto
postcards, then sort these into piles according to classification.

The purpose of all this is to get at the underlying meaning of the situation
for respondents, to see what concepts lie behind the answers they gave, the
events you saw. At the beginning of this chapter we said that there were
different approaches to the use of qualitative data and the approach will
dictate the depth of analysis undertaken. If you are just starting out in
research, probably the most straightforward and useful way of analysing
such data is to try to develop your own interpretation and explanation of
how things are.

It could be that your literature search provided a framework that supports
your findings and places them into a theoretical context that explains or
clarifies the particular research question you are attempting to answer. If
you started out to test a particular hypothesis, the data analysis will be for
the purpose of supporting, refuting or modifying that hypothesis.

Glaser and Strauss (1967) are generally regarded as the most prominent
proponents of what is known as 'Generating Ground Theory'. This means –
in its simplest form – looking for theory to explain the data in the data itself,
rather than looking to existing theory into which the data have to be 'fitted'.
Once concepts begin to emerge and a tentative theory has been formulated,
the researcher returns to the data to test the theory out and to see how the

theory must be modified to fit the data that has been gathered. Further data are then collected, but this time only those that are relevant to the theory generated. Data collection and analysis is thus a sequential process.

Whatever method and approach you choose to analyse your data, you should continue to scrutinise the material until you feel that no new concepts, ideas or interpretations are left. The theory or framework that you are using for your analysis should explain all of your data. If there are some things that seem to contradict this, ask yourself why this is. 'Deviant cases', that is instances that are different to the rest, should not be ignored. By attempting to understand why certain respondents or situations are atypical, you may reach a fuller understanding of the way in which the analysis explains the data and of the theoretical interpretation.

SCENARIO

So how is Student Nurse Green to proceed? Given the limitations of time and expedience, participation in a closed context is probably the most suitable method. The ward has a system of patient allocation, so Student Nurse Green thinks that by observing how patients she is allocated behave and what they say while she is caring for them, she will be able to pick out the features that relate to their operation and treatment, and to find out how they feel about what effect this will have on their lives after discharge.

There could be a problem with recording data, but as nurses are forever writing things down on charts and care-plans, Nurse Green hopes that this will be possible without being too obvious to patients. She will, however, have to look at these records as soon as she goes off duty to make sure they are as complete as possible before she has forgotten what she observed. Recall falls off sharply with the passage of time. Student Nurse Green will also be able to record what patients ask the doctors on the ward round, sit in on case conferences and discharge meetings, look at medical and nursing notes and record which other agencies are brought in, such as the social work department.

Student Nurse Green intends to analyse the data sequentially, so as the study proceeds the data she collects will become more focused and directed to particular concepts as they emerge, checking and refining her ideas, or exploring difficult or 'deviant' cases of patients who seem to have different views to those most commonly expressed.

Although Student Nurse Green will be attempting to generate theory from the data itself, she will need to make use of established theory as a background to the work and to give her some clues as to the sort of attitudes she is likely to find. Otherwise she will be going into the research blindfold and could take a long time in making sense of what she finds going on around her.

BIBLIOGRAPHY

Davis F (1963) *Passage through Crisis*. Indianapolis: Bobbs-Merrill Co. Inc.

Dingwall R and McIntosh J (eds.) (1978) *Readings in the Sociology of Nursing.* Edinburgh: Churchill Livingstone.

Field P A and Morse J M (1985) *Nursing Research: The Application of Qualitative Approaches.* London: Croom Helm.

Fox D J (1976) *Fundamentals of Research in Nursing,* 3rd edn., ch. 12. New York: Appleton-Century-Crofts.

Garfinkel H (1967) *Studies in Ethnomethodology.* Cambridge: Policy Press.

Glaser B and Strauss A (1967) *The Discovery of Grounded Theory: Strategies for Qualitative Research.* Chicago: Aldine Publishing Co.

Hughes J A (1976) Getting involved. *Sociological Analysis: Methods of Discovery,* ch. 5. Walton on Thames: Thomas Nelson.

Krausz E and Miller S (1974) *Social Research and Design.* London: Longman.

Macleod Clark J and Hockey L (1979) *Research for Nursing: A Guide for the Enquiring Nurse.* Aylesbury: H M and M Publishers.

Moser C and Kalton G (1979) Methods of collecting the information – 1. 'Documents and observation' and 3. 'Interviewing'. *Survey Methods in Social Investigation,* 2nd edn., chs. 10 and 12. London: Heinemann Educational Books.

Munhall P L and Oiler C J (1986) *Nursing Research: A Qualitative Perspective.* Conn: Appleton-Century-Crofts.

Oppenheim A N (1966) *Questionnaire Design and Attitude Measurement.* London: Heineman Educational Books.

Potter J and Wetherall M (1987) *Discourse and Social Psychology.* London: Sage.

Treece E W and Treece J W (1986) 'The interview' and 'Observation'. *Elements of Research in Nursing,* chs. 17 and 19. St. Louis: C V Mosby.

9

Ethical Issues in Research

Ethics is a word often used in nursing, but just what is it? What is the definition of ethics? Probably no two people would define it in exactly the same way, but their answers are likely to have common features. The Concise Oxford Dictionary defines ethics as:

> Relating to morals, treating of moral questions, morally correct, honourable.

Cassell's English dictionary says:

> Treating of or relating to morals, dealing with moral questions or theory, conforming to a recognised standard.

How we interpret the concept of moral values will be dependent on the society in which we live. In western societies cultural mores determine the rights of the individual. The way these are respected is fundamental to the way the wider community can be judged.

In looking at the way this philosophy relates to nursing research, the first question to ask must surely be 'who constitutes the community?' You might try discussing this in class or with colleagues to find out how different people interpret the concept of 'community'.

For the purposes of this chapter let us consider three constituents:

1. The researcher.
2. The respondents.
3. Societal context.

It is all too easy to see each of these elements as having separate ethical needs. However, a little thought will reveal that this is not the case. A nurse may be a researcher in one situation, but a respondent in another, and nurses are themselves members of society. The rights and wrongs and moral duties and obligations, then, are common to all. It is the perspective by which these terms apply that changes according to the role of the individual in the research context.

Rights and wrongs, duties and obligations in any society must be based on the values of that society. In western civilisation these values tend to concentrate on individuals and their right to be treated as of worth. No doubt we will each have values that others would not share, but those most likely to be held in common will emphasise this aspect of respect for individuality. How can this be applied to research in general and nursing research in particular?

THE RIGHTS OF THE INDIVIDUAL

1. Not to be harmed.
2. Self-determination.
3. Privacy.
4. Confidentiality.
5. Self-respect and dignity.
6. To be able to refuse to participate at any stage of research.
7. Not to be refused services.

We can look at each of these in turn to see just what they mean.

Not to be harmed

This encompasses all forms of distress: physical, psychological and emotional. It is fairly straightforward to see how physical distress might be caused by some forms of research, but less obvious regarding psychological or emotional trauma. Just think, however, about the way respondents chosen because they had cared for a terminally ill relative at home might feel if asked how they felt about their situation or what were its worst aspects. Distress could also be caused if respondents were asked to face feelings or attitudes, perhaps about themselves, which they preferred to ignore.

Self-determination

Self-determination is more complicated than it looks at first glance. What it means in practical terms is that respondents should only give 'informed consent' to participate. But how can you tell them everything about the research as this may well influence the results? The answer is that information given should be as honest and accurate as possible, but if it is not possible to reveal the full facts of the methodology of the research, it is best to state this, but undertake to explain this after the data have been collected.

Privacy

Privacy is of particular concern during some forms of data collection, such as observation – is it unethical not to tell people they are being observed, whether directly or by the use of mirrors, cameras or tape-recorders?

Confidentiality

The amount of information now kept about each of us by different agencies, much of it on computer, makes this a particularly difficult issue. If you promise confidentiality, you must stick to this. The consequence of this, of course, is that it is impossible to follow up interesting questionnaires or similar research instruments where confidentiality was promised, and some way of compensating for this should have been built into the research design or recognised and accepted at the outset. Some researchers have cheated by using elaborate techniques such as the positioning of stamps on envelopes or some other mark, but this is unethical.

Self-respect and dignity

Clearly respondents should not deliberately be made to look foolish. This includes the right not to be deceived.

To be able to refuse to participate at any stage of the research

Consent will, of course, be sought before any data collection takes place, but it is very hard on the researcher if respondents say they wish to withdraw once a study has commenced. Nevertheless, it must be made clear that they are at liberty to do this.

Not to be refused services

Services, such as treatment or health care, should not be dependent on agreement to participate. Such a condition constitutes pressure, so consent has not been freely given.

VULNERABLE SUBJECTS

There are some groups of people who are not always able to stand up for their own rights, which has ethical implications when the research is concerned with such groups or where the sample may include these people.

Write down the people you feel could be classed as 'vulnerable' in this sense.

You will probably include the following in your list:

- Children
- Mentally ill or mentally handicapped
- The aged
- Captive persons
- Dying, sedated or unconscious persons
- The very poor, who may be dependent on certain services

The consent of parents, guardians or other legally responsible persons should be sought for the participation of those not capable of making their own decisions. The degree of freedom of captive persons and perhaps those in the Armed Forces to refuse participation is debatable. Even where consent is given for or by any of these vulnerable subjects, the researcher is still ethically bound not to take undue advantage and abuse their rights.

The whole question of ethics in nursing research was considered so important that in 1977 the Royal College of Nursing issued guidelines for nurses undertaking or associated with research. These cover nurses undertaking research, nurses in positions of authority where research is carried out and nurses practising in places where research is being carried out. As a profession, nursing must adhere to ethical principles in relation to research and to be seen to do so. As a discipline relatively new to research, nursing must demonstrate that its cherished role as a caring profession does not stop short as soon as it enters a field where issues are far less sharply defined and where the temptations to expediency are great.

THE ROLE OF ETHICAL COMMITTEES

In order to oversee the ethical issues in research in health care, every health district has an Ethical Committee. Universities and other institutions also have Ethical Committees. Their actual constitution and terms of reference may differ from place to place, but the principles will be the same. The role of health district Ethical Committees is to ensure that the research that is conducted within that district does adhere to an ethical code, in particular that the rights of the subject are preserved and that subjects are protected from possible harm. Every research project that involves patients in any way should be submitted to the committee for approval prior to its commencement. Just what constitutes a research project is not always clear cut, but any investigation on man raises ethical issues, whether it is invasive (doing something to respondents) or non-invasive (use of case records, etc.) Research can also be classified as:

1. Therapeutic, which may benefit the respondent; or
2. Non-therapeutic, which is unlikely to benefit the respondent directly.

Both have ethical implications.

As the vast majority of research coming before such committees is of a medical nature – drug trials or new forms of treatment – the emphasis tends to be on medical research. However, the obligation to gain consent for research applies equally to nurses and other health-care workers, and an increasing number of the projects being submitted for approval to health district Ethical Committees nowadays concern research from disciplines other than medicine.

It is not strictly speaking the responsibility of most Ethical Committees to decide upon the scientific merit of the subject, design or implementation of the studies brought before it. However, it would clearly be unethical to give approval to research over which the members had serious reservations and various arrangements are made to cope with this eventuality.

The membership of such committees may well differ from district to district, but a typical health district Ethical Committee will probably consist of members of the medical staff of consultant status, a general practitioner, a member of the Community Health Council, a member of the health authority and a senior nurse. There may also be someone from the legal profession. If the health district is one that has a university in the area that has some association with health-care teaching or research, there will probably be at least one member from the relevant university faculty.

Ethical Committees of other organisations will obviously have a role that reflects the needs of that particular institution, and the membership will be selected accordingly. Though the specific roles may differ, all Ethical Committees serve much the same function and operate on similar principles.

Submission to an Ethical Committee has to be on a formal protocol document, several copies usually being required. Every Ethical Committee will have its own protocol, but as most of the applications are to do with research from a medical or scientific discipline, the protocol is likely to be very detailed and heavily scientifically oriented. This can make it rather difficult for nurses undertaking research to complete. It is a good idea to seek the advice of a nurse whom you know has made an application to such a Committee or to seek the help of the secretary of the Ethical Committee to whom you are making your application.

Whatever the actual format, the protocol will ask certain questions:

1. *Researcher's name and appointment.*
2. *Title of project.*
3. *Objective (or hypothesis).*
4. *The benefits you expect to result from the project.*
5. *Study design.* A brief description of what the researcher intends to do, e.g. administer a questionnaire to patients attending out-patients' departments. A copy of any research tools should be attached to the protocol.
6. *Scientific background.* For nurse researchers this is likely to be a very brief outline from the literature e.g. 'Jonson (1984) demonstrated that patients made a satisfactory recovery following herniorrhaphy performed as day-surgery. Madlow (1985) found that community nurses expressed positive attitudes towards caring for patients who had undergone day surgery. No work to date has examined the type or duration of care required by such patients following discharge, or their attitude towards this approach to surgery.'
7. *Whether the investigation has been done before, i.e. by others.* It could be a replication, which is acceptable, or that you are conducting the

research in a different setting, or using a different sample or some other modification.

8. *If so, why do you wish to repeat it?* This is not a problem as long as you are clear about this.
9. *How many subjects you will require.* That is, how big is your sample?
10. *Whether this size sample is statistically viable.* If your research is of a statistical nature then you would need to state the statistical advice you had received.
11. *How you intend to select them.* There must be a rationale for the selection. Opportunism won't do.
12. *Whether the use of an animal model has been considered.* This is usually not applicable to nursing research.
13. *Invasive procedures to be carried out on patients.* This is usually not applicable to nursing research.
14. *Samples required, e.g. blood, urine.* Also usually not applicable.
15. *How you will go about data collection.* E.g. 'Patients will be given a letter explaining the project and asking for their participation at the first post-operative visit. If they agree, a questionnaire will be administered at that and the subsequent three visits by the community nurse. Approximately 20 minutes will be required for completion on each occasion.'
16. *Discomfort likely to be experienced by subjects.* This may seem to be another non-applicable question, but consider the psychological effects your research may have.
17. *Hazards or harm to subjects.* The same considerations as above.
18. *The precise information to be given to subjects.* Either the letter of explanation should be quoted or a copy attached to the protocol.

Ethical Committees may meet monthly, or every 2 months. The application for ethical approval is, therefore, a vital factor in any research timetable, as data collection cannot proceed without it. Not getting an application in on time could result in a delay of 3 months before the project can continue, so it is worth finding out about this well in advance of the date you wish to start collecting data.

Exercises

1. Write down the questions you would want to ask, if you were approached for your consent for your 9-year-old child to take part in research into children's attitudes to violence.
2. List the ethical problems that our ward team must consider.

In a group you could organise a role play in which one member of the group acts as a researcher trying to gain the consent of ward nurses on whom it is intended to conduct non-participant observation of the nature of the nurse–patient interaction, without disclosing the subject of the research.

SCENARIO

The ward team seek the advice of a tutor from the diploma course who has carried out several research studies as to whether they need to apply to the district Ethical Committee and how to go about this.

The tutor suggests that as it is a team project that involves a variety of research methods and will take some time to complete, they should discuss the proposed research with the Ethical Committee's secretary. The tutor considers that as Sister Jones' research will be concerned with examining past records and hospital statistics, she will not need to seek the Committee's consent for this individually as it is non-invasive. There would, of course, be considerations of confidentiality to remember if she had intended to look at patients' case notes. Staff Nurse Baker does not need ethical consent either for her experimental research on nursing records as these are regarded as an internal matter and patients will not be directly involved in the data collection. Sister Brown, on the other hand, intends to question patients and their relatives as part of her research, so for this phase of her investigation will need to make an application to the Ethical Committee. Student Nurse Green wishes to carry out closed participant observation, directed at the feelings patients express with regard to discharge following surgery. Although this is a non-invasive technique, and patients will not be affected in any way, Student Nurse Green must bear in mind that she has a duty to respect any confidential matters she may hear and be careful to ensure that her records are kept in a safe and secure place.

There are two other aspects to this question of ethics that the team must remember. First, they have a duty to seek the permission of their manager to carry out the research. It is the manager, after all, who will be ultimately accountable should there be a complaint or some similar difficulty. Second, although the team is conducting nursing research, the medical consultant has responsibility for patients, so discussion with the relevant consultants is not only a matter of courtesy but also their agreement is vital if the research is to succeed.

BIBLIOGRAPHY

Ashworth P (1984) Accounting for ethics. *Nursing Mirror*, **158** (10): 34–36.
Bulmer M (ed.) (1979) *Censuses, Surveys and Privacy*. London: Macmillan.
Cassell's English Dictionary (1966) London: Cassell.
Concise Oxford Dictionary (1976) Oxford: Oxford University Press.
Diers D (1979) *Research in Nursing Practice*, ch. 12. Philadelphia: J B Lippincott.
Macleod Clark J and Hockey L (1979) *Research for Nursing: A Guide for the Enquiring Nurse*, pp. 6–11. London: H M and M Publishers.
MacMillan M (1981) A view of ethics. *Nursing Times*, **77** (18): 786–787.
Royal College of Nursing (1977) *Ethics Related to Research in Nursing*.

Royal College of Physicians (1984) *Guidelines on the Practice of Ethical Committees in Medical Research.*

University College Hospital Ethical Committee (1981) Experience at a clinical research ethical review committee. *British Medical Journal,* **283** (6302): 1312–1314.

P J Verhonick and Seaman C S (1982) Ethical issues in nursing research. *Research Methods for Undergraduate Students in Nursing,* ch. 5. New York: Appleton-Century-Crofts.

10

Data Analysis

If, as we have argued throughout this book, research is a problem-solving process, then analysis of the data helps to see if we have the evidence to solve our problem, to answer our question. At the end of any research study we are faced with a mass of undigested data. Data analysis techniques are simply a means of organising or summarising the data to look for patterns and order. This applies whether you have used quantitative or qualitative data collection methods. In the first case you have numbers, and in the second words, but systematic approaches are needed in both cases to make sense of the data.

Systems for analysing qualitative data have already been described in Chapter 8. This chapter will be concerned with quantitative data and statistical approaches to analysis. The approaches we will be discussing would apply to data from experimental or survey research studies.

Many people find this the most off-putting stage in research, probably because of a fear of maths that survives from school. When you have some results from your own research, however, statistical techniques can appear less threatening. They are, after all, common-sense tools to bring some order out of chaos, and you do not have to be a mathematical genius to use them. We do not regard ourselves as mathematical geniuses, just people who have gained understanding through coping with our own data and becoming more confident with practice. We therefore feel able to appreciate the level of difficulty that other people experience when confronting data analysis and offer our own coping strategies. You could call this a 'Mickey Mouse' guide to statistics! It is correct, but we have tried to make it as straightforward and understandable as possible. There are plenty of exercises to learn techniques and gain confidence.

DEFINITIONS

The word 'statistics' has more than one meaning. It can mean:

- The data themselves
- The activity of analysing the data
- Specific statistical tests

and we shall be exploring all of these aspects, in that order, in this chapter. We shall, therefore, be talking about statistics at two main levels: the level of *interpreting* data (research reports and official statistics), and the level of *doing* statistics.

OFFICIAL STATISTICS

Official statistics can be a valuable source of information in research in several different ways:

1. You can consult the various digests of statistics as part of your literature search (see Chapter 3) for baseline information on the population to be studied. For example, in a study within psychiatric nursing you might want to quote the annual rate of admission and discharge of patients to long stay hospitals over a given period.
2. Reading official statistics can often generate ideas for research – puzzling patterns and connections between things that you would like to explain in more detail. An example might be the connection between health and occupation or class that is published in official statistics tables.
3. The figures themselves can also be analysed further in a quasi-experimental study (see Chapter 6 on experimental methods). Studying figures before and after a change in law or policy, say community care policies, could yield new insights into the effectiveness of that change.

Exercise

Write down as many types of official statistics as you can think of.

Discussion

You are likely to have thought of the census, which is the most comprehensive means of collecting data in Britain, but there are various forms of data collection used by the government. They can be categorised in the following way:

1. *Census.* Data on households collected nation-wide every 10 years. Useful baseline data, although it can be several years before all the results are published.
2. *Rating records.* Registers of electors.

3. *Vital registration*. Births, deaths, marriages, divorces.
4. *Surveys*.
   - Continuous (annual/bi-annual – 10 000 per annum): general household survey; family expenditure; national food survey; labour force survey; new earnings survey.
   - Ad hoc, e.g. women's employment; family formation; national dwelling and housing; industrial relations; Royal Commissions, etc.
5. *Administrative structures*. E.g. DHSS – hospital bed-days, number of doctors, prescriptions; Chief MOH Report; crime statistics; unemployment; education.

Most of these statistics are the by-product of the book-keeping data of various government departments published for general use. For an index or guide to possible statistical sources of information in your area of interest consult the *Guide to Official Statistics* published by the CSO (Central Statistical Office). Perhaps the most digestible form of government statistics comes in publications like *Social Trends* and *Population Trends* from the CSO that will be available in most libraries. These are published yearly and summarise data from many sources with useful commentary and discussion. The topics include population, housing, environment, education, employment and income, as well as health and social services information.

Official statistics do need to be approached with some caution, however. There may be problems associated with the collection of the data that need to be taken into account in interpretation.

There might be *technical* problems such as a high non-response rate, which biased the sample. The terms used might not have been defined consistently over time. For example, the census definitions for bathrooms changed over time so it is difficult to see if there is any real change in people's living conditions.

Other problems might occur with the *meaning* of terms and categories. What are the assumptions and values behind the statistics? Who selected the categories? Who defined the terms? Apparently 'hard' data such as cause of death can, in fact, be decided with some discretion by doctors, police and coroners.

ANALYSING VARIABLES

When it comes to *doing* statistics we would suggest a simple procedure to guide you. You can 'ease' yourself gently into a set of data by following this series of steps:

$$\text{Data} \longrightarrow \text{Table} \longrightarrow \text{Graph} \longrightarrow \text{Statistics}$$

These steps will be demonstrated through exercises in the rest of the chapter. The procedure is the same whether you are analysing one variable or more. The statistics can increase in level of complexity and sophistication. We will mostly be concerned with *descriptive* statistics, deriving figures that *describe* patterns in the data. The majority of nursing research studies report results at this level. Some use *inferential* statistics (i.e. the statistics are used to infer, say, a causal relationship between variables) and more advanced statistical procedures such as *regression analysis*. Our treatment of these methods will be more at the level of interpretation – how to interpret this kind of result when you encounter it in a research report.

Exercises

The following exercises are based on the step-by-step guide outlined above. You can apply them to your own data and data will be given. Most could be done 'by hand' but you might prefer to use a calculator. In practice, if you were involved in a research project, a computer program could do all the calculations you need in minutes, but it helps if you understand the process first.

Data

Exercises

(Answers are given at the end of the chapter.)

1. Let's start by generating some real data on which to practise. How much sleep do you get compared with other people? Jot down as accurately as possible the times you went to bed and the times that you got up, to the nearest half-hour, over the last 7 days. Then collect the same information from a few other people, say members of your family or colleagues at work, noting in addition their sex, approximate age and any other details that you think are interesting. We should point out at this stage that this exercise is for demonstration purposes only and will not follow strict statistical rules such as sampling.

    We could start summarising the data by seeing on how many occasions people went to bed by midnight or had more than 8 hours' sleep. To do this count up the total number of bedtimes or nights of sleep from all the people in your sample (this should be the number of people multiplied by seven, for the number of days you are covering). Now count the number of occasions you are interested in, whether it is bedtimes by midnight or more than 8 hours' sleep. To compare the people who went to bed later or had less sleep, you simply calculate the remainder from your total. An example is given at the end of the chapter.

2. The results can be made even clearer by converting the raw data to percentages because this puts the results on a standard scale and

makes comparisons easier. To convert your data into a percentage, make a fraction from the occasions of interest over the total and multiply by a hundred. For example:

$$\frac{\text{bedtimes by midnight}}{\text{total bedtimes}} \times 100 = \% \text{ bedtimes by midnight}$$

An example is given at the end of the chapter.
3. Now try summarising some data collected in a survey of perceptions of health. Respondents were asked:

'Do you think you should make any changes in your life-style to benefit your health?' (Yes or No)
177 said Yes and 69 said No. Express those numbers as percentages. The answers are given at the end of the chapter.

Tables

The next step in our step-by-step procedure is to express our results in table form. In the example above we would present the numbers as we have in Table 10.1:

Table 10.1   Frequency table of bedtimes data – 1

Bedtimes	Number
By midnight	24
After midnight	11
Total	35

This type of table is called a frequency table – in other words a table that shows how frequently certain categories occur. With only the two categories of answer, such as Yes and No, it is usually enough to quote the results in your report without needing a table. When you have several categories of answer it becomes more necessary to communicate the results through a table.

A frequency table would be useful if we wanted to summarise our data by bedtimes or hours of sleep, from the earliest to the latest, the longest to the shortest, etc. Notice in our example in Table 10.2 that it is usual to give both the raw figure and the percentage.

Table 10.2 Frequency table of bedtimes data – 2;
Table to show hours of sleep per night

Hours	Number	%
6–7	10	28
8–9	16	46
10–11	9	26
Total	35	100

Exercises

4. In the survey of perceptions of health, the respondents who felt they should make changes in their life-style were asked which area of change was a priority:

   54 answered 'exercise', 28 'relaxation', 61 said 'diet', 24 'to give up smoking', and 10 'To cut down on alcohol'.

   Construct a frequency table, including percentages, for the data. An answer is given at the end of the chapter.

Graphs

The tables in all our examples could next be translated into graphic form, such as a bar chart, histogram or pie chart. The advantages here are that the human eye and brain seem to assimilate information more easily in visual form. If a graphic display does not communicate results more clearly than text or table, it has not been properly used.

Figures 10.1 and 10.2 show the data from Table 10.2 converted into bar chart and pie chart form. Both illustrate how much more effective a graph can be than a table in communicating results.

Exercises

5. Try converting your data to charts and compare with our examples.
6. Draw a pie chart from the table in Exercise 4 (above) for priority areas for change in life-style (see table in Answer 4 at the end of the chapter). The answer is given at the end of the chapter.

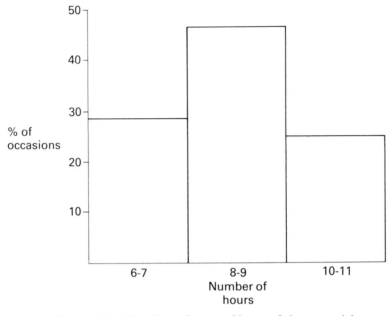

Figure 10.1   Bar chart of range of hours of sleep per night.

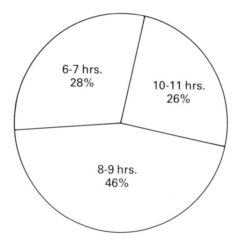

Figure 10.2   Pie chart of range of hours of sleep per night

Statistics

Data that have been presented in table or graph form can in turn be summarised by just one or more statistics.

Averages

The first summary statistic that is usually calculated is an *average*. There are three different types of average to choose from, largely depending on the type of measurement that was used:

1. *Mode*. The value that occurs most often (the most common value).
2. *Median*. The value that is exactly half way in the order of values (the central observation).
3. *Mean*. The sum of the value of all observations divided by the number of observations.

The mean is the average most familiar to us from schooldays and everyday calculations, but it is not always the most appropriate. For example, it was once quoted on a current affairs programme that the average salary is £20 000. This may be a sore point, but the majority of us do not seem to approach anything like that figure in our annual salary. The point is that it does not take many salaries of £100 000 or higher to distort the average if you are calculating a *mean*. Commonsense suggests that it might be more accurate to find a figure that the majority of us receive (the *mode*) or some figure half-way along the scale from the lowest to the highest (the *median*).

Exercises

7. Calculate the *mode* from the following set of salaries:
   £6 000
   £8 000
   £10 000
   £10 000
   £10 000
   £12 000
   £12 000
   £14 000
   £16 000
8. What is the *median* for this set?
   £6 000
   £12 000

£18 000

£24 000

£30 000

9. And the *median* for this set?

£6 000

£7 000

£9 000

£13 000

£15 000

£15 000

10. What is the *mean* here?

£8 000

£10 000

£12 000

£14 000

£16 000

11. Which average do you think most appropriate for the bedtimes data?

Discussion

We have already shown in the bar chart in Figure 10.1 that 8–9 hours is the usual amount of time for sleep. This is the mode and probably the easiest and most sensible summary statistic for this data. In fact, if we calculated the median and the mean we would also come up with somewhere between 8 and 9 hours.

As a general rule of thumb, use the mode with a simple set of data like this, as the most commonsense way of expressing an average. With a larger and more complete data set, the median is a very reliable average, but if you are likely to be applying statistical tests then calculation of the mean will be necessary.

A more technical explanation is that the choice of average depends on the level of measurement of the data. The mean can only be used with 'continuous data', i.e. measures in order on a continuous scale such as salary or temperature (also called parametric data). With 'discrete data' (or non-parametric data) the mode or median are more appropriate. This is where the measures are in discrete categories and not in numerical order, for instance different professions or days of the week.

Exercise

12. Would you express the average of the perceptions of health data in Answer 4 as a mode, median or mean?

Discussion

Once again, with this type of discrete data, the mode is the commonsense choice because one would want to say that, on average, more people mentioned diet as a priority for change in life-style.

Standard deviation

If data are continuous and could be represented on a graph as a smooth symmetrical curve, then all the data can be summarised by just two statistics – the mean and the standard deviation. The standard deviation is a measure of the shape and distribution of the data represented by the curve and shows by how much the scores deviate from the mean. It is the most commonly used measure of variability in data. It is useful for locating an individual score relative to others and in comparing samples.

If, for example, we measured the heights of a large section of the adult population and mapped these on to a graph, we would arrive at a shape something like that in Figure 10.3.

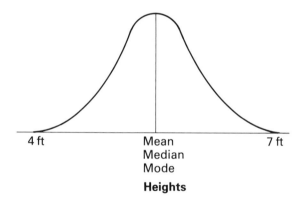

Heights

Figure 10.3   Normal curve for measures of height

This is like a smoothed-out histogram and it is the typical symmetrical or 'normal' curve that has been observed for measures of human characteristics. There is a large range of measures, with a large proportion of them around the central observation. In the example of height, the measures range from 4–7 ft, but the majority are around the 5 ft 5 in mark – the average.

We should point out that the word 'normal' has a precise technical meaning here and is not used in its usual sense in nursing. The notion of a normal distribution is fundamental to the statistics of sampling, where some sort of estimation or probabilities are involved. Probability statistics will be discussed later under the heading of 'Inferential statistics'.

As Figure 10.3 shows, in a normal curve the mean, median and mode averages are identical and fall at the central point. If the curve were 'skewed' or had more than one peak, the mean, median and mode would probably differ. The median would be a more reliable indicator, but the mean would be needed for statistical tests. Most statistical tests, however, assume that the measures follow a normal curve.

Figure 10.4 shows that on a normal curve the first standard deviation falls at the point either side of the centre where the curve changes shape.

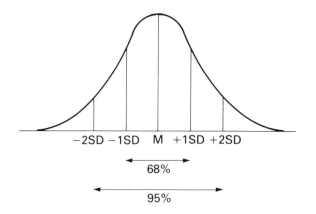

Figure 10.4　Normal curve for IQ measures showing standard deviations

The standard deviation is a more accurate way of expressing the curve than a measure of range because it is not so influenced by extreme values at either end of the curve. In the example of heights if one or two people were over 8 ft tall this would give a false impression of the range.

The standard deviation is useful in statistics because it conforms to certain rules. From Figure 10.4 it can be seen that 68% ($\frac{2}{3}$) of the observations in the curve fall between one standard deviation either side of the mean and 95% between two standard deviations either side of the mean.

These regularities in data can be used to predict and plan services and are the basis of disciplines such as community health. The principles are applied in the field of educational testing, for instance, where IQ tests such as the 11-plus exam have previously been used to stream children in secondary education. If the mean IQ were 100, children with a score higher than one standard deviation above the mean at 115 would be considered grammar school material. Those $2\frac{1}{2}$% achieving above 130 or two standard deviations would be considered gifted.

At the other end of the scale, children and adults scoring less than 85 or one standard deviation below the mean on an IQ test have traditionally been labelled as mentally handicapped. The $2\frac{1}{2}$% below two standard deviations were seen as severely mentally handicapped. From such percentages it has been possible to calculate the incidence of severe mental handicap in the population and plan the size of necessary provision and services.

Calculating the standard deviation

As we said earlier, the scope of this chapter is more the interpretation of statistics. If you need to calculate standard deviations for your own data, we suggest you consult a statistician or one of the references listed at the end of the chapter.

TWO OR MORE VARIABLES

In this chapter we have suggested a simple procedure for analysing data, forming this series of steps:

Data ⟶ Table ⟶ Graph ⟶ Statistics

As we shall now demonstrate, the same procedure applies when you are analysing more than one variable.

Data

It is a good idea to start with a list of questions that you want to ask of the data. Your original hypotheses or research questions should be the starting point. You might want to verify, for instance, whether there was a difference in results between different ages, between men and women, etc.

Tables

When you are cross-checking categories of more than one variable, you can organise the frequencies of the data into a *contingency table* (also called cross-tabulation).

To continue the example of the survey on perceptions of health, we might be interested in whether there was a difference between how men and women answered the question 'Do you think you should make any changes in your life-style to benefit your health?' The contingency table in Figure 10.5 shows the breakdown of Yes and No answers by gender.

A computer program would produce a table like this from your data in a flash. If you have to do your data analysis by hand, you are limited to rather more labour-intensive methods, like sorting all your questionnaires into two piles – one for men and one for women – and then counting how many in each pile said Yes and how many said No.

Notice how in Figure 10.5 converting the raw figures into percentages helps to highlight the relative proportions of the groups, especially if there

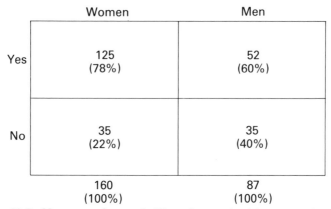

	Women	Men
Yes	125 (78%)	52 (60%)
No	35 (22%)	35 (40%)
	160 (100%)	87 (100%)

Figure 10.5 Necessary changes in life-style perceived by men and women

are uneven numbers in the groups. In this case there were almost twice as many women as men. This was not a biased sample, however. As it was a sample of nurses it was fairly representative of the population.

If there is a pattern in the data, this should be revealed in the table. In Figure 10.5 does the pattern of response differ between men and women, that is, as one set of responses increases, does the other set decrease? In this case there does seem to be a tendency for women to say they will change their life-style more than men, although more than half of both groups were willing to change.

We can demonstrate the process of cross-tabulation with an example from the bedtimes data. Let us start with the raw data in Table 10.3, and ask the question: Is there a difference between teenagers and adults in the amount of sleep they have?'

Table 10.3 Hours of sleep of a small sample of people over a week

Person	Age	Mon	Tue	Wed	Thu	Fri	Sat	Sun
A	44	6	7	6	7	8	8	7
B	40	7	7	6	7	6	8	8
C	17	9	9	8	7	10	10	8
D	15	9	9	8	9	10	11	8
E	13	10	10	10	10	9	9	9

The table can be constructed by tallying the different amounts of sleep over the week, between the two groups, as shown in Figure 10.6:

Age group Hours	Adults	Teenagers	
6-7	~~HHT~~ ~~HHT~~	I	11
8-9	IIII ،	~~HHT~~ ~~HHT~~ II	16
10-11		~~HHT~~ III	8
	14	21	35

Figure 10.6 Tally of differences in amount of sleep between teenagers and adults over a week

The final table appears in Table 10.4. Is there a difference between teenagers and adults?

Table 10.4 Differences in amount of sleep between adults and teenagers over a week

Hours	Adults	Teenagers	Total
6–7	10	1	11
8–9	4	12	16
10–11	0	8	8
Total	14	21	35

Exercise

13. Try a contingency table on your own bedtimes data. As well as age groups you could compare men and women, see if there was a difference in bedtimes or hours of sleep between weekends and weekdays or use any other interesting variables.

Graphs

Variables measured by continuous or parametric scales can be plotted on to a graph in a *scatter plot*. For example, we might hypothesise that there is a relationship between length of service and salary, both of which are on a continuous scale and could be plotted on to a graph to see whether there is a link. It could be that both variables will increase, as one goes up so does the other. Or that as one goes up the other goes down. Or that there will be no connection at all. In the fictitious example in Figure 10.7 it does indeed look as though salary increases with longer service!

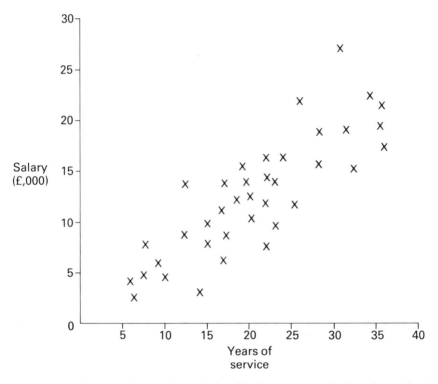

Figure 10.7   Scatter plot to show relationship between length of service and salary

The variables of age and hours of sleep used in the contingency table in Table 10.4 are also continuous variables, even though we divided them into two (a *dichotomy*) or three groups for the table. We could plot the data on to a graph and look for a pattern. If there is one, it should show even more clearly in a scatter plot. The trend should be that the older the person, the less sleep he or she gets. There are not really enough cases over a wide range of ages in our data set, however, to get a true pattern.

Exercise

14. Try a scatter plot on your own bedtimes data. Have you enough observations and a wide enough age range to see a definite pattern?

Statistics

The statistic for summarising data in frequency tables with more than one variable is called the 'chi-squared test' (or χ^2). Because it is used with discrete groups or categories in tables, it is a non-parametric test. It assesses whether there is a pattern or link between the variables in the table, and, therefore, helps to test hypotheses. In Table 10.5 we have shown the data from Figure 10.5 together with the chi-squared statistic, which should help us to decide whether there is a difference between men and women's views on changing life-styles for health as hypothesised. The chi-squared test has been used with a 2 x 2 table here, but can be used with larger tables.

Table 10.5 Necessary changes in life-style perceived by men and women, with chi-squared statistic

	Women	Men
Yes	125	52
	(78%)	(60%)
No	35	35
	(22%)	(40%)
Total	160	87
	(100%)	(100%)

Chi-squared = 7.85

The principle behind chi-squared is to test whether differences in the data in a contingency table are real or just due to chance. If they are 'real', the hypothesis is supported, and we can say we have a 'statistically significant result'. 'Significance' is used in this way, not in the everyday sense of 'important' or 'remarkable', but in a narrower statistical sense that will be discussed more fully in the next section.

The figure of 7.85 in our example is the result of the chi-squared equation. This figure must in turn be checked against a table for the chi-squared test to see if it is statistically significant. The figure is, in fact, significant, which means that the table shows a link between gender and attitudes towards change in life-styles. In other words, we have some sound evidence for the hypothesis that women are more likely to say they will make changes in their life-style for the sake of their health.

We do not need to go into the details of the calculations of the chi-squared test here. You can get that from the references at the end of the chapter. As we have said before, it is more important in the first instance to be able to interpret such statistics when you encounter them in nursing studies.

Inferential statistics

The chi-squared test is an example of *inferential* statistical tests that *infer* the probabilities that the results from your sample are typical of the population as a whole. The results of tests like this are often expressed in a probability statement. You may have read studies which said something like: 'significance level $p < 0.01$' or 'the results were statistically significant at the 0.05 level of confidence'. This means that no more than once (0.01) or five times (0.05) in a hundred would you get these results if chance factors alone were operating. You can, therefore, be 99% (0.01) or 95% (0.05) confident that the results were due to your intervention, your independent variable. In other words you can accept your experimental hypothesis and reject the null hypothesis. It is a bit like the odds for betting in horse racing.

0.01 and 0.05 are the usual levels for accepting significance. With most data 0.05 is acceptable, but if you need to be cautious, the level should be set at 0.01 or even 0.001. In clinical trials, for instance, you would need to be very sure that treatment was effective before introducing it into practice, especially if there were possible harmful effects. The lower the probability value, the more confident you can be with the results.

Some computer programs for data analysis will print out a probability value to compare with the levels of statistical significance. In a study of student nurses' attitudes, for example, the value given for differences in attitudes between the beginning and end of the course was $p = 0.04$. You can see that it is statistically significant because it is below the $p < 0.05$ level and, therefore, lends support to the hypothesis that training will influence nurses' attitudes.

The chi-squared test is used to describe contingency tables. *Correlation statistics* are needed to describe the continuous variables that would be represented in a scatter plot. Correlation means the degree or amount of association or similarity there is between two variables. A correlation coefficient expresses this amount as a number between 0 and 1. The most commonly used procedure produces a correlation coefficient called r. If the r value is high, say 0.8, it means that the two variables are closely related; if the r value is low, say 0.1, it means that the two variables are not closely related; if the r value is negative, e.g. -0.8, it means that the two values are negatively related (i.e. the greater the one, the less the other).

For example, in a survey of people's drinking patterns a correlation coefficient of 0.6 (a positive correlation) was calculated between people's normal intake and the amount they drank at Christmas. As one figure increased so did the other. The trend therefore suggested that the light drinkers drink lightly at Christmas and the heavy drinkers drink heavily at Christmas. In another example, when people were asked how interested they were in exercise, a negative correlation was found between the rate of interest and their age, so that the older they were the less interested they were in exercise.

In your reading, you may encounter the terms r^2, R and R^2, which are part of regression analysis. Regression is concerned with the nature of the relationship between continuous variables but is a rather advanced statistical procedure for this chapter. Guidance to doing or interpreting these sorts of statistic can be found in the references at the end of the chapter.

Correlation tests are available for use with either continuous or discrete data. The parametric test is called the Pearson Product Moment Correlation, the non-parametric test is the Spearman Rank Order Correlation.

To choose the right test you need first to decide whether parametric or non-parametric measures were used in the data. Parametric means that the data must conform to *parameters* or rules for use with particular tests, such as type of measurement, normally distributed data, random sampling and the same standard deviations for the samples being compared.

If in doubt use the non-parametric test. It is less powerful and more cautious than the parametric test. You are more likely to get non-significant results, but if you do show significance then you probably have a real result.

The same rules apply when you are choosing a statistical test to check the results of an experiment for significance. The various inferential tests have been developed to try to assess the difference between experimental groups and conditions, to see whether the independent variable has an effect as hypothesised.

If two different groups or approaches are being compared under the same conditions, such as our washing-up liquid experiment in Chapter 6, then the t-Test (independent samples) is the appropriate parametric test, whereas the Mann-Whitney U test is the one for non-parametric data.

If you are comparing the same group of people or matched groups under one or more conditions, as in the example of comparing different teaching methods in Chapter 6, the parametric test is the Matched Pairs t-Test, and the non-parametric test is the Wilcoxon Matched Pairs Signed Rank Test.

More details of the use of these tests and others are in the references at the end of the chapter.

COMPUTERS

We have hinted several times at the tremendous advantages of using a computer package to help with your statistics and strongly reommend that you seek advice on this. Don't be daunted by the technology because the computer can do your calculations in a fraction of the time it would take by hand or by calculator. It is not necessary for you to learn how computers work or to learn computer programming or languages. You only have to learn how to use one of the ready-made statistical packages available for personal computers and on larger computers (e.g. SPSS).

Three of the nurses in our research team on Ward 4 have generated data for analysis from their individual projects.

Sister Jones has been looking at admission lists for surgery to calculate the likely effect on Ward 4 of the change in policy to short-stay. She had also offered to gather data on referrals for Sister Brown.

Sister Brown, the community nurse, has collected data over 2 months on the time spent by community nurses with surgical patients. Later on she will have to process the results of her main survey on how patients and carers cope at home.

Staff Nurse Baker has been comparing the number of times two different types of nursing process notes were used on the ward.

We are not going to discuss all of the results, but we can use some of them for more exercises.

Exercises

15. Table 10.6 is a table that Sister Jones has compiled to show the surgical admission lists for the hospital over 4 weeks. She is interested in three groups of patients:

   - Those staying for 1 or 2 days, because this is the group that might in future be treated as day-surgery patients.
   - Patients staying between 3 and 5 days. If this group are to be treated as 5-day patients in future, there will be implications for admission. Patients could only be admitted for 5-day stay at the beginning of the week. Admissions later in the week would have to be allocated to another type of ward.
   - Long-stay patients, that is patients staying more than 6 days would also have to be allocated to a different ward, or be considered for 5-day stay. The issue here is that patients would have to be screened carefully for fitness for short-stay surgery, otherwise the work-load for the community nurse would be greatly increased.

   From Table 10.6 calculate the percentages of patients in each group over the 4-week period. Answers are given at the end of the chapter.

16. Sister Jones's table of surgical patients referred to the community by hospital liaison sisters over 2 months is shown in Table 10.7. Try converting the table into a histogram to show the different proportions of surgical patients from each ward over the 2-month period. What proportion of surgical patients is from Ward 4? Answers are given at the end of the chapter.

Table 10.6 Surgical admission lists for hospital over 4 weeks

Length of stay per week	Number of operations per surgeon (A–E)				
	A	B	C	D	E
WB March 20					
1–2 days	5	1	3	6	7
3–5 days	10	6	10	2	6
6 + days	2	1	4	1	3
WB March 27					
1–2 days	1	5	7	5	5
3–5 days	4	2	8	5	11
6 + days	0	0	4	0	1
WB April 3					
1–2 days	2	4	3		6
3–5 days	7	6	12		6
6 + days	2	0	1		1
WB April 10					
1–2 days		3	6		6
3–5 days		3	8		11
6 + days		0	1		0

Table 10.7 Surgical patients referred to the community over 2 months

	Hospital liaison referrals (surgical)	
Ward	March	April
1	3	1
2	11	12
3	17	15
4	10	11
5	2	2
Total	43	41

17. Table 10.8 shows the data collected for Sister Brown by community nurses of visiting times to surgical patients. If you remember, the data

were recorded over 2 months on the forms shown in Figures 7.22 and 7.23. Fill in the final blank column by calculating the mean time for visits per patient. How would you interpret these results? Answers are given at the end of the chapter.

Table 10.8 Visiting times of community nurses to surgical patients

Ward	No. of patients	%	Average age of patients	Actual time all patients	Average time per patient
1	24	28	44	47h 15m	
2	30	36	49	26h 15m	
3	21	25	44	26h 15m	
4	4	5	64	43h 15m	
5	5	6	45	13h 00m	
Total	84	100	46	156h 00m	

18. For her study on the use of the new nursing process notes compared with the existing notes, Staff Nurse Baker developed a check-list of criteria to check whether the different stages of planning had been completed satisfactorily. She found that all 30 patients admitted to her experimental group had full and comprehensive care plans.

In the control group, where the existing notes had been continued, less than 50% of the 30 patients had complete care plans. Although the care given was well documented, the stages of assessment, planning and evaluation were often partial and inadequate.

Staff Nurse Baker wants to use a test to see if there is a statistically significant difference between the two groups. Which statistical test would be appropriate? Answers given at the end of the chapter.

BIBLIOGRAPHY

Cormack D F S (ed.) (1984) *The Research Process in Nursing,* chs. 14, 15 and 16. Oxford: Blackwell.
Goldstone L A (1983) *Understanding Medical Statistics.* London: Heinemann.
Huff D (1973) *How to Lie with Statistics.* Harmondsworth: Penguin Books.
Knapp R G (1978) *Basic Statistics for Nurses.* New York: John Wiley and Sons.
Polit D and Hungler B (1983) *Nursing Research: Principles and Methods,* chs. 14, 15, 16 and 17. Philadelphia: Lippincott.
Reid N G and Boore J R P (1987) *Research Methods and Statistics in Health Care.* London: Edward Arnold.
Robson C (1977) *Experiment, Design and Statistics in Psychology.* Harmondsworth: Penguin Books.

Rowntree D (1981) *Statistics Without Tears*. Harmondsworth: Penguin Books.
Treece E W and Treece J W (1977) *Elements of Research in Nursing*. New York: C V Mosby.

ANSWERS TO EXERCISES

1. People in the sample had 8 or more hours sleep on 24 out of 35 occasions. 11 of 35 bedtimes in a week, therefore, were less than 8 hours.
2. 69% of bedtimes in a week were by midnight, 31% were after midnight.
3. 72% said Yes. 28% said No. (To calculate the percentage each figure was divided by the total of 246 and multiplied by 100.)

4. Table: Priority areas given by respondents for change in life-style

Area of change	n	%
Diet	61	35
Exercise	54	30
Relaxation	28	16
Smoking	24	13
Alcohol	10	6
Total	177	100

6. Pie-chart of priority areas for change in life-style:

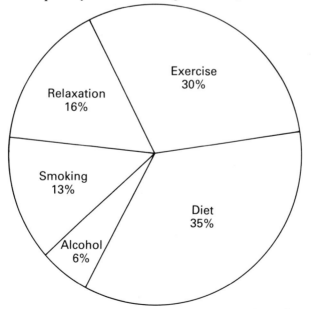

(Note: the different areas could be shaded or coloured to contrast)

7. £10 000 is the mode, because it occurs most often.
8. £18 000 is the median because it falls half-way in the order of values.
9. £11 000 is the answer. As there are an even number of figures, you need to calculate the mid-way point – in this case between the third and fourth value.
10. The mean is £12 000.
11–14. Answers can be found in the Discussion sections in the text.
15. There is a total of 213 patients over the 4 weeks. Each group expressed as a percentage of that is:

	%	n
1–2 day patients	35	75
3–5 day patients	55	117
6 + day patients	10	21

16. To design the histogram, you need first to total the figures for 2 months for each ward and then convert these to percentages. The table with converted figures would look like this:

Table: Hospital liaison referrals for surgical patients March/April

Ward	n	%
1	4	5
2	23	27
3	32	38
4	21	25
5	4	5
Total	84	100

From this, it can be seen that 25% of surgical patients are from Ward 4. The pattern is clearer still in the histogram.

17.

Ward	No. of patients	%	Average age of patients	Actual time all patients	Average time per patient
1	24	28	44	47h 15m	1h 58m
2	30	36	49	26h 15m	0h 52.5m
3	21	25	44	26h 15m	1h 15m
4	4	5	64	43h 15m	10h 49m
5	5	6	45	13h 00m	2h 36m
Total	84	100	46	156h 00m	1h 51m

To calculate the mean time for visits per patient convert the actual time for each ward into minutes. For example:

Ward 1: $(47 \times 60) + 15 = 2835$ minutes

Then divide the figure by the number of patients:

$$\frac{2835}{24} = 118 \text{ minutes (rounded figure)} = 1 \text{ hour } 58 \text{ mins}$$

There are some interesting differences here. The most striking is an average time of 10 hours 49 minutes per patient for surgical patients from Ward 4. The column for average age of patients seems to give a clue. In fact, Sister Brown discovered that the figures for Ward 4 were distorted by one patient who was aged 93, taking 30 hours of day-nurse time, and 10 hours of night-nurse time. Although it was the patient's wish to be at home, Sister Brown questioned the disproportionate amounts of community nurse time involved. The figures are also an indication of the wide variation in community nurse input which would be influenced by changes in surgical policy.

The findings do not really relate to age but to dependence. Sister Brown had assumed that there would be a relationship between age and time taken but various statistical tests produced no significant results.

There is a variation in average time per patient between all the wards. Sister Brown concluded that these needed explaining by further investigation of medical records. It could be that different wards had different admission policies or dealt with different kinds of surgery.

18. The choice of test would, of course, depend on the type of measure Staff Nurse Baker used. It is likely that the measures would be discrete – for example, simple Yes/No categories or a check-list of criteria for the completion of stages in the nursing process. If she scored each stage on a rating scale of say 1–5, however, the data might be treated as continuous. Generally speaking though, it would be safer if she chose a non-parametric test. Since she is comparing matched paired groups under two different conditions (the use of new notes compared with existing notes), the correct non-parametric test is the Wilcoxon Signed Rank Test.

11

Communicating Results

TYPE OF REPORT

One of the problems with much nursing research is the difficulty of communicating the results of studies to the rest of the profession. This is in part because not all nurses make the effort to read research articles or reports.

Nevertheless, only by writing up and publishing their studies can nurses who conduct research add to the body of knowledge in nursing. It could be argued that they have a positive duty to do this and so hopefully stimulate debate upon the subject from others. This does, of course, mean that one's work is open to comment and criticism, but this is surely what must happen if nursing is truly to become a research-based profession.

Professional development is only one of the reasons for writing reports and publishing articles. The other reasons that may or may not be applicable in any given situation are:

Reporting back to the funding body

If the research has been funded in any formal way, most organisations will request a report at the end of the study. Even if they do not, it is only courtesy to provide some feedback so that the organisation can see how their money was spent, the findings which emerged and what benefits may have come about.

Request for further funding

On long-term research, a report may be requested at the 'half-way' stage and the continued funding may be dependent on the results up to this point. Alternatively, if the research has been successfully completed but further research is indicated, a good report can help either in approaching the original funding body, or in seeking the support elsewhere.

Informing colleagues

Research is a disturbing and challenging affair, not just to the researcher. Colleagues may well have had to cover some duties, swap days off or even take messages for the researcher. Whatever the circumstances, no research takes place in a vacuum and colleagues will inevitably have been affected in some way. Informing them just what it was you have been doing all this time and what it is you have found out is not only a courtesy, but also shows them that their co-operation was valuable and worthwhile. If the research was conducted in the work-place, they clearly need to know about the findings and the implications for practice.

Providing feedback to participants

Participants may, of course, have been colleagues. However, they might well be people you do not expect to be in contact with again. For some, a full-scale report would be unsuitable, but you do have a duty to inform those who have agreed to take part in a research study just what was found. Quite what form this takes will depend on the situation, but to ignore the need is arguably unethical.

HOW TO GO ABOUT IT

Inevitably some people are more gifted than others in writing research reports or articles fluently and clearly, but the task can be made simpler by following the basic rules and working through systematically. In fact, that is the key to successful writing: simply follow the steps of the research process and even if your style lacks polish the report or article will be effective and readable.

One important thing to remember is that how and what you write will depend on the intended audience. The kind of report that would be prepared for a funding organisation would not be appropriate say, for colleagues on a ward, or for a journal, and might be different again to participants. However, the same areas need to be covered. What needs to be communicated is:

1. Why the study was conducted.
2. How the study related to previous work in the field.
3. How it was done.
4. What the results were.
5. Where you go from here.

These points form the sections into which a report is conventionally divided. To put this more formally, the report should contain an introduction, a review of relevant literature, an explanation of the methodology, explanation of the results, and finally a section discussing the results, and the conclusions and implications of the findings.

There are four steps to writing a report:

1. *Preparation*. This is when you think through the purpose of the report and identify the audience who will read it, checking for accuracy and collecting facts and ideas from different sources. You should start to make notes under the sub-headings of the report.

2. *Arrangement*. What sequence is the convention for your particular field? Select a title that is informative but not verbose. Select the information you will use, being ruthless about rejecting irrelevant material. Then revise and decide on the order. Separate files or a card index may help. Put the material under the headings you have chosen, adding extra notes as required. Decide whether or not there will be appendixes, illustrations and so on, and how you are.going to arrange these.

3. *Writing*. Write clearly and simply. Using flowery language or 'jargonese' will not make your report seem more learned, in fact quite the reverse. The purpose after all is to communicate.

4. *Revising*. Give yourself time for this. It is a good idea to put the draft on one side for a few days, then go back to it again. Make sure the pages are numbered correctly, that diagrams and appendixes are labelled and that references are complete and accurate. Getting someone else to read it through can be helpful.

So just what should go in each section? Although the actual contents will vary according to the particular circumstances, below is a guide to the things you need to take into account.

Introduction

A report or paper has to be written as if those who read it will know little or nothing of the subject. Of course, this is rarely the case in practice, but the point is that you must not assume that people will automatically know what you mean unless you tell them. So the introduction has to set the scene as it were, explaining how the research came about, in what way you were involved in that field and the importance of the research with regard to current practice. Why is it of interest to you or anyone else? The introduction has to explain the context of the research and to convince the reader that it is worthwhile reading on.

Literature review

The nature of the literature review will depend in part on the audience for which you are writing. If the paper is an internal report or to a funding body, then it might not be appropriate to give an extensive review of the literature unless you are requested to do so. Nevertheless, some discussion of previous work on the subject and the different theories which form part of current thinking on the subject is necessary if your paper is not to appear trivial and lacking in depth. You will need to be rigorous in deciding just what literature is central to an understanding of the subject. This is a very good discipline in writing pithy but useful reports!

On the other hand, should the paper be intended for publication, or be part of the requirements for a course of some kind, the literature review could well take up a quarter to a third of the entire paper. This is because you will need to provide a much fuller discussion concerning previous work, the varying theories that may have been argued and the literature that led you to the formulation of your hypothesis and theoretical framework. This is not just writing for the sake of it – if you wish to persuade the readers that your research has been meaningful, you must demonstrate that your work has been conducted in the light of, not ignorance about, other research on this topic.

Methodology

It is important to explain precisely how you went about the study, just what form your data collection took. The things to include in this section are:

1. What method of data collection was used; a questionnaire, observation, interviews or whatever. If you are writing for publication, it is not feasible to give the whole of your research instrument – the complete interview schedule for instance. But you can include one or two items as examples. In a full report or large-scale piece of research it is the convention to give the whole of the instrument in the form of an appendix at the end.
2. Why you chose this method instead of others. As we said in the chapter on research design there is no 'right way' to conduct research, so you need to explain the thinking behind the method you adopted. What led you to reject alternative approaches? What were the advantages and disadvantages of the methods you rejected, and just as important, what were the advantages and disadvantages of what you did do? What problems were encountered in the research and how were these overcome? Would you do the research in the same way with the benefit of hindsight?
3. How the sample for research was chosen, and how respondents were contacted and their consent obtained. If there are ethical implications or difficulties, these should be discussed, and the decisions made justified.
4. The arrangements made for the analysis, whether this was manual or by computer. The results themselves come in the next section, but

you should explain how the analysis was carried out and if help was given by anyone else. If, for example, a statistician actually put the data onto a computer and ran the analysis for you, or assisted you in doing it yourself, you should state this.

Results

It is easier for others to read if results are presented separately from the discussion about their interpretation, but it may not be easy to do this in a limited space. However, try to avoid a jumble of tables, graphs, lists of numbers and so on all mixed up with the text on what they mean. The chapter on data analysis will have given you some ideas on how to present data in a clear and methodical manner. One graph can be worth a hundred words, so think who your readers will be, and whether they will be able to understand what you are showing them. Obviously, only the most important results can be presented in an article where the number of words is limited, but other papers should contain all your findings. Again, if these are extensive, then some could be put in an appendix.

DISCUSSION, CONCLUSION AND IMPLICATIONS

Having presented your results, you should discuss just what they mean. It is all very well to state that in answer to Question 14, which was about pre-operative anxiety, 20% of patients answered 'very', 60% answered 'quite' and 20% said 'not at all', but what does that mean for practice in surgical nursing, and how does it relate to the question about previous admission to hospital for example? More importantly, what are the implications for practice in the future? The recommendations you may wish to make concerning change should follow logically from the discussion, supported as that is by the results. It is often said that all research does is come up with more questions, but that should not be regarded as a criticism. Once you begin to investigate an issue you are more likely to discover that there is more to it than you first thought, and further research is necessary. It would be an unproductive piece of work if it led nowhere!

PRESENTATION

So what should this report look like? For a start it should be attractive. That does not mean that it has to be on glossy paper, but it should be neat and tidy. Handwritten reports or articles are not acceptable, but the advent of word processors means that it is easier these days to get your work in typed format, or you could get someone to type it for you. A report such as you would write for a sponsoring body should have the following:

Title page

This should include the name of the author and the date.

Acknowledgements

You will have been helped on your way by numerous people, and it is only courteous that you should thank them in a public manner. You don't need to name them all individually, but something like:

> My thanks to the Royal Elephant Society who funded this work, to the computer section at Hightown College of Further Education who gave valuable advice on the analysis, and, not least, to my colleagues in Ward 4 for their support and encouragement.

List of contents

This should contain the headings of the various sections and the number of page on which they start. It makes for easier reading if each section starts on a fresh page and each page should be numbered. There should also be a list of tables or figures, giving the label of each one and the page number. If you have any appendixes, these should be listed, stating what each is and again giving a page number. Conventionally, appendixes are given roman numerals, e.g. 'Questionnaire page ix'. This distinguishes the appendix from the main text.

Summary

The summary should do just what the name implies, i.e. summarise the work. A large report will probably have a summary of 200 words, a more modest piece of work would only require a sentence or two, e.g.

> A study was conducted on fifty patients following herniorraphy to investigate their experience of community care after discharge. Whereas the majority considered their needs to have been met, a significant number felt they would have benefited from greater involvement with the Community Nursing Sister. Changes in the liaison system following surgery are recommended.

Chapters or sections

Appendixes

List of references

In the text you will only have referred to other work as 'Jones (1)', or 'Jones, 1987'. The list of references would then be listed in numerical order or alphabetically:
1. Jones B C (1987) *Nursing for Students.* London: Blackstock Publications.
2. Smith A B (1986) *Community Care.* Manchester: White Publishing.

Make sure your references are complete and correct. If you were careful enough to record them as you went along then you should have no problems but, if not, you are in for a frustrating time searching them out again!

WRITING FOR PUBLICATION

The most important point in getting your work accepted for publication is to submit it to the most appropriate journal in the first place. Consider the topic of the research and ask yourself what kinds of people would be interested in reading about it. It could be suitable for one of the 'popular' nursing journals, but if it is very specialised or for a particular speciality in nursing – community nurses, say, then the journal that caters for that particular group of nurses would be best.

Most journals have guidelines for contributors to help in the preparation of articles submitted for publication. If you cannot find this in back copies of the journal in question, it is worth writing or telephoning to ask for these to be sent to you. In general, journals will ask for manuscripts to be double-spaced with a margin of 1 to $1\frac{1}{2}$ inches. You should send the original manuscript, not a photocopy, but remember to keep at least one copy for yourself. Length will vary according to the journal, but 1,500 to 2,000 words is about right for most publications. You could telephone or write to the most appropriate journal, saying you have an article on so-and-so and would they be interested in publishing it. This will save a lot of time if they are not publishing the kind of material you are offering, so you can then apply elsewhere.

Much of what has already been said about writing reports applies to writing for publication also, but there are some particular points to bear in mind.

1. The content and style will depend on the intended readership. It is useful to read several copies of the journal you intend to submit your work to in order to get a 'flavour' of the articles the journal publishes.
2. The title of the paper needs to be particularly clear and concise and accompanied by a statement of who you are.
3. The literature you discuss and references you give should be those that are most central to the research. References should be presented in the convention adopted by the particular publication to which you intend to submit your article. There simply isn't space for everything you read that had some bearing on the topic or the way it was investigated.
4. Only an outline and the purpose of the methodology should be given. Again, detailed explanation is not possible or appropriate.
5. Choose the tables and figures you present with care. Limit these to findings that demonstrate the most crucial results. Remember, some people may only read your work in journal form, so get across the most important points.
6. There should be some discussion of the implications of the results, though of necessity not extensive, but it will probably not be appropriate to give recommendations too except in general terms, as these are specific to the setting in which the work was conducted.

7. The limitations of the work – what you would do or not do again, unexpected difficulties encountered and ways in which the research could have been improved should be stated. This is not just 'washing one's dirty linen in public'! It demonstrates that you are fully aware of any faults and have considered them both for your own benefit and for research on that topic in the future. Besides, it is better to admit one's shortcomings or mistakes than have others point them out later!

8. As with reports, it is usual to acknowledge those who have helped in the research or gave permission for it to be conducted.

Exercises

1. From the information we have given in the various chapters, try writing the introduction for a report on Ward 4's project that will be presented to the Unit General Manager.

2. Put yourself in the place of one of our ward team, and write the section on research design and methodology for an article to be submitted for publication to one of the nursing journals.

3. Look for journals that would be suitable for an article on Ward 4's project and make a short-list. Find out the name of the person to whom you should send it. Then write a letter to this person, stating what the article is about, and asking if they would be interested in publishing it.

These exercises can be done individually, but with a group of colleagues or in class could then be compared for content, clarity and style.

BIBLIOGRAPHY

Abdellah F and Levine C (1979) *Better Patient Care Through Nursing Research*. New York: Macmillan.

Cheadle J (1984) Presenting your research. *Nursing Mirror,* **146** (18): 26–28.

Darbyshire A E (1974) *Report Writing*. London: Edward Arnold.

Notter L (1979) The research report: communicating the findings. *Essentials of Research in Nursing,* ch. 10. London: Tavistock Publications.

Polit D and Hungler B (1985) Research reports. *Essentials of Nursing Research,* ch. 19. Philadelphia: J B Lippincott.

Seaman C H C and Verhonick P J (1982) The student's report: organisation and self-evaluation. *Research Methods for Undergraduate Students in Nursing,* ch. 16. Conn: Appleton-Century-Crofts.

Tierney A (1984) Writing and publishing a research report. *The Research Process in Nursing* (ed.) D F S Cormack, ch. 17. Oxford: Blackwell Scientific Publications.

Treece E W and Treece J W (1986) 'Writing the research report' and 'Publication of the research report'. *Elements of Research in Nursing,* chs. 25 and 26. St Louis: C V Mosby.

Ward R A (1977) *100% Report Writing*. Thames Polytechnic.

12

Writing a Research Proposal

The ward team are understandably proud of their efforts so far. As is usual in most fruitful research, they realise that there is a lot more that could be done to develop the project further and, after some discussion, decide to apply for funding to extend the work. In order to do this they are advised by the tutor from the school of nursing that they will need to write a research proposal.

Writing a research proposal is a very useful procedure, which can contribute much to the success of any research project. It is not just a requirement for funding applications.

REASONS FOR WRITING A PROPOSAL

So what is the purpose of a proposal? Well, the proposal can serve a number of purposes.

First, if you are seeking funding in order to undertake the research, the proposal is necessary to explain to the body being approached just what is intended. The proposal, and the way in which it is prepared, will help to demonstrate that you have thought through the research carefully, appear competent to conduct the work and are clear as to just what you are proposing to do.

Second, writing the research proposal is an excellent way to clarify one's thoughts. A proposal is like a blueprint, and in preparing it you will have to be specific as to the nature and purpose of the research. Writing the research proposal is the crucial event that turns a collection of woolly ideas and vague hopes into a realistic exposition of intent.

Third, a good proposal serves as a guide in writing the report at the end of the study.

Fourth, if you are conducting the study as part of the requirements for a degree or some other form of higher education, a research proposal may well be required by the department at the university or college with which the researcher intends to register. Indeed, acceptance for registration is usually dependent upon the quality of the research proposal.

The research proposal should cover three things:

1. Why the study should be done.
2. How it is to be conducted.
3. What will be the benefits of completing the study.

STYLE

In most cases when researchers apply for funds the research proposal has to be submitted to the funding body to examine, before deciding whether or not even to interview the applicant. Therefore, it has to speak for you, it has to 'sell' the idea on its merits.

Sometimes a funding body or other organisation may issue guidelines on just how a proposal should be set out. It is a good idea to emphasise those aspects of the research that you consider will be of particular relevance to that specific organisation. Although the research will probably have been discussed with a lecturer if further education is involved, the same considerations apply. It goes without saying that the proposal must be convincing. If it is rather vague, those reading it will question whether you are really competent and committed.

Equally obviously, it should look good. A neat, well-organised, clear proposal will carry far more weight than a bundle of dog-eared papers that are hard to read and understand.

STEPS FOR PREPARATION

It is worth following the steps listed below before you actually complete the proposal. This will help to ensure that all the major aspects have been covered.

1. Write down the study objective and research questions to achieve that objective as clearly as possible. Do not try to put the world to rights in one go! You will only end up with confused objectives and numerous overlapping questions.
2. Review the literature. This will, of course, be part of the research process, but demonstrating a knowledge of previous work in the subject and how your proposal relates to this will show that you have given the matter some thought.
3. Plan your overall design. Decide whether the approach is to be survey, experimental or interpretative. The objectives of the study will probably indicate the most appropriate design. Then you can work on developing the research tools.
4. Decide to which funding agency application will be made. Some

agencies may have their own proposal protocols, so the proposal will need to be prepared in the required format. Some information on funding agencies is given at the end of the chapter.

5. Seek a 'mentor'. If this is your first attempt at research, the advice and support of someone more experienced will be invaluable and save many pitfalls. Even experienced researchers discuss their plans with colleagues, so do not feel embarrassed about seeking help. Find out if the health district has a research adviser or if there is a research interest group. The Royal College of Nursing has a full-time research adviser who can probably provide a local contact for you.

6. Think through what it is you hope the eventual analysis will look like. With quantitative data, the tables, charts and so on that may result are fairly easy to speculate on, but it is more difficult to imagine the form of qualitative data. The point of the exercise is that it will shed some light on the quality of the data you can expect to collect and, therefore, whether it will prove worthwhile.

7. Be brief but clear. Funding agencies and other bodies are not likely to be swayed according to the weight of the documentation before them. Indeed, as they often have many such proposals to read they are likely to be less enthusiastic over considering one of daunting proportions!

8. Keep supporting papers brief. Just what is included in a proposal in the way of appendixes may be laid down by the agency. If not, ask yourself if the intended appendix is relevant and necessary. If it is not, then leave it out.

9. Realistically assess the required resources. If the intended research will require the use of a computer and you have no access to one, how do you propose to overcome this? How much time will the research really take and will you be able to get this time out from work?

10. Cost the research carefully. Find out how much it will cost to type and photocopy the research tools you plan to use. What will the postage be? What mileage rate is reasonable for travel? It is much better to get this right before you send in a proposal than to run out of money before the research is complete. The agency will not be too keen to consider a request for further funding if this happens.

Figure 12.1 presents the things you need to think about when writing a research proposal in the form of a flow chart.

CONTENTS OF A PROPOSAL

As previously discussed, some bodies have specially prepared proposal forms, and though they will differ from one another, they will all be likely to include the following:

Stages of research	The bright idea / The predicted problem	What shall I be reporting? (← A) → The research question(s)	Measures / Procedures	Sample	Data collection and analysis	Further questions → Return to A
Methodological questions	What do I know about relevant methods?	For what alternative explanations must I control?	Construct validity? Ecological validity? Internal validity? Reliability?	Population validity? Internal validity?	Will the data be sufficient to answer the question? Will they be sufficient to reveal alternative explanations I have not considered? Will they be in a form amenable to analysis?	What other material could I collect using the same resources?
Ethical and political questions	Whose interests are involved in this area? What are the main problems?	Who would be threatened by the questions being asked? Who would *feel* threatened by the questions being asked? Does my phrasing of the question, or my selection of the topic, prejudge the problems?	Is there a risk of damage or embarrassment to subjects? Is deception a necessary part of the procedures? Confidentiality?	Is any group excluded who ought to participate?	Will they be sufficient to cover the problems? Will they be sufficient to allow an alternative explanation to be argued by interested parties?	What is the likely effect of my conclusions on research subjects? What is the likely effect of my conclusions on other interested parties? What additional data shall I need to counter possible objections?

Figure 12.1 Constructing a research proposal. (Reproduced with permission from Open University, Course DE304, Research Methods in Education and the Social Sciences)

Title

The research proposal must have a working title, even though it is possible that the emphasis of the research may shift as it proceeds. Try not to make the title too long, although it should make clear just what the subject of the research is.

Name of the investigator

This sounds too obvious to need saying, but the point is you need to ensure that your name is clearly written on the document itself, not just on the accompanying letter that went with it, which can become separated from the proposal.

Date of submission

This looks equally obvious, but if the research lasts 2 or 3 years and you were committed to completing it within a certain time scale, there should be a record of precisely when it was started.

Statement of the problem

Here it must be stated clearly just what research problem you are studying. The proposal is most likely to succeed if this problem, although specific to the area of your enquiry, has more general application. A research problem that was only of relevance to a particular clinical area and had no application to similar settings is unlikely to gain support. The problem should be of a manageable size, given the resources at your disposal and the time scale envisaged. The problem can be in the form of a hypothesis or it can be expressed as a question that it is intended the research will attempt to answer.

Importance of the problem

Is there really a requirement for research into the problem you have identified? It may be of interest to you, but is anyone else likely to think the same? Who will benefit from the work? Will there be implications for further research? If there is a theoretical basis for the study or if it will contribute to previous theory, this should be discussed. You may consider that the research will contribute new theory to the field of knowledge on the subject, in which case discuss how this might come about. Is the project unique, or has the same or similar work been done before? This would not rule it out as long as you can make a case for repeating it or can demonstrate the singular feature of what is proposed.

Objectives of the study

What is it you are setting out to achieve? The objectives should be realistic and they should relate to the problem as it has been outlined. The objectives that are stated should be specific and they must be measurable. 'To improve nursing care' will not do!

Precis of the literature

The proposal should contain a résumé of the relevant literature. This should be aimed at presenting an overview of the subject or topic to be studied. Past studies of particular interest and the strengths and weaknesses of these should be discussed, demonstrating how the research being proposed will explore these problems. The literature review might pick out suggestions or leads for further research suggested by other researchers, and present a synopsis of the results of past work. The literature should be as up to date as possible, emphasising current research.

Research design

The proposal should state, first, what approach it is intended to pursue – survey, experimental or interpretative. Second, the hypothesis to be tested or the research question to be investigated should be clearly stated. Third, the definitions you intend to use, the limitations of the research and the assumptions being made must be clearly set out.

Research implementation

Although at the proposal stage it is not usually expected to include prepared questionnaires or other research tools, you should have some idea how the required data will be collected, what kind of data you intend to collect and the facilities necessary for the analysis. This latter point is particularly true if the analysis will be dependent on computer facilities and advice. The approving body will want to be sure that you have made or are making arrangements for this and that the research will not grind to a halt because you overlooked the problem of analysing a large volume of data.

Resources

If the proposal is being written in order to apply for funding for the research, it must state how much money will be required and how it will be spent. Travel associated with the research, the cost of printing or photo-copying data sheets, questionnaires or other research tools, typing, postage, must all be included here. The timetable is another factor, especially where the funding request is of a major nature and includes the salary of the researcher or research team.

SCENARIO

In order to extend the research, the ward team are requesting financial support to enable Staff Nurse Baker to continue with the project as part of her staff-development course. The amount of money being sought is, therefore, fairly modest, as it is only intended to cover research expenses. The research proposal they finally draft is shown below:

Implications for nursing practice of day- and 5-day surgery

Susan Baker, Registered General Nurse. Intensive Therapy Certificate. Senior Staff Nurse, Ward 4, Hightown General Hospital. 12 September 1989.

Background to the study

The increase in day surgery and the utilisation of 5-day wards is a policy that has become more and more widespread in the last 10 years. It is stated DHSS policy to encourage this form of treatment in order to reduce waiting lists[1]. The costs per patient treated are also less, and there is some evidence that such treatment is more convenient and well accepted by patients.

Whereas 5-day wards have been in operation for some time in this country[2], the needs of these patients have received little attention.

The District Health Authority intends to introduce a 5-day ward undertaking minor general surgery in the next financial year. The aim of the research is to:

1. Examine the precise care needs of patients treated on the new ward.
2. Determine the most effective and efficient way of meeting these needs.
   The findings would hopefully be of relevance not only to the proposed facility but also to other 5-day units.

Literature review

Day-surgery is not quite the modern innovation in patient care that it is often assumed to be. Nicoll[3] published the first account of day surgery in 1909, and considered that patients experience less pain and have a lower incidence of respiratory and circulatory complications.

Burn[4] states that as the cost per patient is less, more patients can be treated using the same facilities. However, in a survey in 1980 of 30 Health Districts who had 5-day units, Davies et al[5] found that 13 of the units were an addition to pre-existing facilities, the aim being to reduce waiting lists.

Ruckley et al[6] suggest that community nursing staff welcomed the variety of patients that day- and 5-day surgery brought into their case-load.

Little research so far appears to have approached the question from the point of view of the patient. What kind of information would be most appropriate both before and after discharge and what are the special care needs of such patients while in hospital?

Research design and method

The research is in two stages.

1. It is intended to visit several hospitals around the country that have 5-day units in order to study their policies and procedures.
2. The criteria by which patients will be selected for 5-day surgery have already been established by the Surgical Division. Using these criteria, patients from the waiting list will be randomly selected to take part in a survey aimed at defining what pre- and post-operative information they consider would be helpful. The project will be explained to them verbally and by a printed description, at the out-patients' clinic. If consent to take part is given, patients will be interviewed at home on an agreed date.

Sample

One hospital from each of 6 different health regions will be visited for the first part of the research. A sample of 60 patients will be randomly chosen for the survey. This size sample has been chosen so that, assuming a 50% response rate, the sample will still allow some statistical analysis.

Analysis

Data from visits to other hospitals will be examined for examples and indications for good practice. The patient survey will be analysed qualitatively for consistent themes in responses to open-ended questions and by computer for the demographic and structured questions.

Ethical considerations

Patients will already have been told of the way in which their operation is to be performed (i.e. day- or 5-day admission) by their consultant, prior to an approach being made. They will be given time to consider participation. Evidence from similar studies suggests that patients welcome the opportunity to discuss forthcoming treatment with a health-care worker. Any difficulties identified will be discussed with the consultant, who has given his support to the study. Measures will be taken to preserve confidentiality of questionnaire responses.

Resources

Hightown College has agreed to undertake the computer analysis of the patient survey results as a student project. The resource requirements, therefore, do not include the cost of analysis.

Travel

Visits to 6 hospitals with 5-day units	£150
Typing of letters to 60 patients	£ 50
Typing and photocopying of questionnaires	£100
Postage	£ 10
Typing and photocopying of report	£ 50
	£360

References

1. DHSS (1976) *Priorities for Health and Personal Social Services.* London: HMSO.
2. Ruckley C V (1971) Team Approach to Early Discharge and Out-Patient Surgery. *The Lancet,* **1**: 177–180.
3. Nicoll J H (1909) The surgery of infancy. *British Medical Journal,* **1909** (2): 753–754.
4. Burn J (1983) Responsible use of resources: day surgery. *British Medical Journal,* **3286**: 492–493.
5. Davies R, Cliff K S and Waters W E (1981) Present use of 5-day wards. *British Medical Journal,* **282**: 2118–2119.
6. Ruckley C V, Ferguson J B D and Cuthbertson C (1981) A 5-day ward as part of a comprehensive surgical service. *British Medical Journal,* **282**: 1525–1528.

SOURCES OF FUNDING FOR NURSING RESEARCH

Department of Health and Social Services

Funds research in health and social services. Responsible for two Research units; Chelsea College at King's College, London University, and Nursing Practice Research Unit, University of Surrey. Awards limited, number of Nursing Research Fellowships annually. Has a Nursing Research Liaison Group and liaison group for social services.

Medical Research Council

Responds to applications from the research community, but unknown territory for nursing research.

Health Education Authority

Funding for educational purposes in health care. Often sympathetic to nursing research if it is educational in intent.

Industry

Pharmaceutical companies in particular fund an enormous amount of medical research. Uncharted territory for nurses, but they are becoming more aware of nursing research.

Economic and Social Research Council

The main funding body for academic research in the social sciences. May be sympathetic to applications related to health care. Provides research studentships as well as research grants.

Regional Health Authorities

All Regional Health Authorities have research funds, which are intended to include funding for nursing research. Most regions also award scholarships or travel bursaries for nurses on an annual basis, but these will be fairly modest in size.

District Health Authorities

Like regions, districts have research funds for employees and sometimes award small scholarships also.

Medical charities

There are a vast number of medical charities, catering for specific conditions. Some are concerned more with patient support services, but most have research commitments also. An untapped source for nursing research, but may well be sympathetic if the research is concerned with their particular interest.

King Edward's Hospital Fund (King's Fund)

This is a type of medical charity, but it has a wide range of activities concerning all aspects of health care, including education, information services and research.

Addresses of all the above can be found in the *Hospital and Health Service Year Book,* which will be found in a hospital or university library.

There are also other guides, such as:

Directory of Grant Making Trusts, published by Charities Aid Foundation, 48 Pumbury Road, Tonbridge, Kent.

Grants Register, published by Macmillan, Basingstoke.

Handbook of British Medical Charities, published by the Association of Medical Charities, London.

Exercise

Think of a project in your own clinical field that you would like to undertake. You could continue with the topic you chose for the third exercise in Chapter 3 if you did that. Then write notes for a research proposal using the following headings:

- Statement of the problem
- Abstract
- Background to study
- Objectives
- Methods
- Work plan
- Personnel involved
- Facilities required
- Budget

FURTHER EDUCATION

Some nurses decide to pursue their interest in research by applying for a degree course. It is not possible here to list all the degree courses available, but they fall roughly into three types:

1. *First degree.* This will lead to the award of Bachelor of Science or Bachelor of Arts. There are an increasing number of degree courses specially designed for nurses, usually for a BSc. Such courses will incorporate the execution of a research project as part of the requirements for the award of the degree.
2. *Higher degree (taught).* A Master of Arts or Master of Science is the 'next level' degree. They may be called 'taught' courses because attendance at formal lectures and other settings is required. However, students are also expected to conduct a fairly major piece of research that will be supervised, but which would be entirely of their own instigation and responsibility.
3. *Higher degree (untaught).* The degree of Master of Philosophy is awarded solely on the research undertaken by the student. This will be supervised, but the student must arrange him or herself to attend

any lectures or seminars. Needless to say, this should only be attempted by those who already have some experience of research, and who have probably obtained a second nursing qualification, such as the Health Visitor Certificate or similar.

Universities and polytechnics will be able to give details of the courses they hold, and the necessary qualifications for entry.

BIBLIOGRAPHY

Brittain R D (1980) Money and methods for research in the National Health Service. *Royal Society of Health Journal,* **100** (3): 79–81.

Daniels N (1974) *Directory of Nursing Scholarships, Bursaries and Grants.* London: Whitefriars Press.

Polit D F and Hungler P B (1985) *Essentials of Nursing Research,* pp. 364–365. London, New York: J B Lippincott.

Salter B (1985) The funding market for nursing research. *Journal of Advanced Nursing,* **10**: 155–163.

Spitzer W (1973) Ten tips on preparing research proposals. *Canadian Nurse,* **69** (3): 30–33.

Treece E W and Treece J W (1986) Design and conduct of the study: proposals and grants. *Elements of Research in Nursing,* pp. 117–122. St Louis, Toronto, Princeton: C V Mosby.

Epilogue

At the beginning of the book we said that research is a 'friendly' activity. We hope that you have discovered that for yourselves now, through the scenario and by working through the exercises, because it is so important for nurses and other health-care professionals to become confident about researching their practice.

Of course there are 'ups' and 'downs' in research. The scenario has given some idea of that. There are usually some dark days in the middle of a research project when things do not go the way you hoped, but the sense of achievement when you overcome such setbacks is tremendous.

Even if you decide you do not want to actually *do* research, hopefully you will be able to share in this achievement by *using* other people's research.

Glossary

Abstract Collection of published research literature that includes a summary of the work.

Action research An experiment in an everyday setting where the researcher introduces change and assesses the outcome(s).

Aim The purpose for which the project was undertaken.

Approach The type of research to be conducted, i.e. survey, experimental or interpretative.

Average A statistic summarising the typical value from a set of data. The three types are mean, median and mode.

Bibliography List of published material, e.g. books, articles, conference papers.

Chi-square (χ^2) A statistical test for checking relationships between variables in contingency tables (non-parametric).

Coding Translating responses to a survey into number codes for processing by a computer statistical package.

Contingency table A table that can show the relative proportions of frequencies of two or more variables.

Continuous data *See* Parametric Data.

Control group A group of subjects in an experiment who are observed under usual conditions to compare with the results of intervention with an experimental group.

Controlled variable A variable that is held constant during research, so that it does not interfere with changes in other variables under study.

Correlation The degree of relationship between two continuous variables, expressed as a correlation coefficient between -1 and $+1$.

Cross-tabulation *See* Contingency Table.

Data Information or facts systematically gathered during research.

Data analysis Techniques that summarise data to identify patterns and order.

Dependent variable The variable that is examined for changes brought about by manipulating the independent variable.

Descriptive statistics Techniques that help to describe patterns in the data.

Discrete data *See* Non-parametric Data.

Empirical A method of testing any hypothesis by a systematically controlled collection of data.

Ethical Relating to moral principles or values.

Evaluation research The systematic collection of information about people, performance and products in order to improve effectiveness.

Experimental research Research that tests an hypothesis by means of a controlled manipulation of variables.

Exploratory research An early stage in some research projects using informal observation and interview methods to refine the hypotheses and research design.

Frequency table A table that shows how frequently certain categories of data occur.

Graph The visual display of data on a chart, e.g. histogram.

Hypothesis A statement that predicts the relationship between variables in a study.

Historical research Research that collects and interprets evidence on past events, sometimes indicating their implications for the future.

Independent variable The variable that is manipulated during the research.

Index Lists of published research articles and papers, often covering foreign language sources as well as English speaking ones.

Inferential statistics Statistical tests that help to make inferences from data, such as causal relationships between variables.

Interpretative research Research that seeks to understand the question under study from the perspective of those participating in the setting.

Main study The major enterprise of the research project, conducted after the pilot study.

Mean   A statistic to average data by summing the values of all observations and dividing by the number of observations.

Median   An average that identifies the value that is exactly half way in the order of values in the data.

Methodology   The methods by which data are collected, e.g. interview, observation. In a wider sense it also means the study of the methods themselves.

Mode   A way of averaging data by expressing the value that occurs most often.

Non-parametric data   Measures in discrete categories and not in numerical order, e.g. different professions, days of the week.

Non-participant observation   A data collection method in which the researcher takes no active part in the situation being observed.

Normal distribution   A smooth, symmetrical 'bell-shaped' curve in a plot of frequency measures. This is necessary if statistical tests are to be applied to the data.

Null hypothesis   A statement that predicts no relationship between variables being tested. This is the basic principle of statistical tests. If tests reject the null hypothesis, this suggests that a relationship does exist.

Nursing research   Research concerned with issues of nursing practice, management or education.

Observation   A method of collecting data by one or more researchers watching and systematically recording the actions or behaviour of those being studied.

Official statistics   The 'book-keeping' data of various government departments, published for general use.

Parametric   Referring to rules or parameters to which data must conform in the use of certain statistical tests.

Parametric data   Measures on a continuous scale, e.g. salary, temperature.

Participant observation   A method in which the researcher is actively engaged in the situation being observed.

Percentage   Data standardised to show incidence per hundred cases.

Pilot study   A small preparatory study usually conducted to test data collection methods.

Population   The total number of people or things in a particular category of interest for study.

Probability   The principle behind statistical procedures that help to assess whether the results of a study show a pattern or occur by chance only.

Project   An activity that seeks to provide information, and which may or may not be empirically based.

Qualitative research   Research in which the data are in the form of words and the analysis aims at identifying underlying concepts and commonly held themes.

Quantitative research   Research in which the data collected are in the form of numbers and which seeks to test the hypothesis by statistical analysis of data.

Quasi-experiment   An experiment conducted in an everyday setting, which therefore does not fully conform to the strict rules of a laboratory study.

Questionnaire   A written list of questions on attitudes, opinions or experiences that is put to respondents. The questions may be administered by the respondent or by the researcher.

Random sample   A sample chosen so that, to eliminate bias, all members of the population have an equal chance of being represented.

Reactivity   Influence of the researcher on the research setting and the data collected.

Regression analysis   An advanced statistical procedure concerned with the nature of the relationship between continuous variables.

Reliability   The extent to which research findings can be generalised to other settings. This can relate to time and place.

Replication   The repeat of previously published research, following the original research design as closely as possible.

Research critique   The critical examination of published research.

Research project   A study conforming to scientific principles and contributing to the body of knowledge of the discipline.

Research proposal   A paper, sometimes formal in structure, that sets out the research question to be examined, the intended design of the study and the expected benefits of the research.

Respondent   The person under study in a survey.

Response rate   The proportion of respondents invited to participate in a study who eventually provide data.

Sample   A sub-set of the population, chosen according to statistical procedures, on which data will be collected.

Scatter plot   Data from two continuous variables plotted in relation to each other on the two axes of a graph.

Semi-structured interview   An interview in which the questions to some topics are open-ended and some are standardised.

Standard deviation   A measure of the variability represented in a normal distribution of data, showing by how much the scores deviate from the mean.

Statistics   This term can mean the data themselves, the activity of analysing the data or specific statistical tests.

Statistical significance   A level at which statistical tests show that results were probably not achieved by chance factors, e.g. 'significance level $p <$ 0.01' means that the probability of the results occuring by chance is no more than once in a hundred.

Stratified sample   A sample chosen to represent specific categories in the population.

Structured interview   A carefully controlled interview in which a set pattern of questions is put to a respondent.

Survey research   Research that seeks to describe and analyse the present situation by means of questionnaires, tests or interviews with a sample of the population.

Table   The representation of data in orderly columns for easier reference.

Theory   A structure that sets out in a formal manner the inter-relatedness of concepts in a particular field of scholarship.

Triangulation   The use of more than one approach, methodology or theoretical framework in a single research enterprise.

Unstructured interview   An interview in which topics pertinent to the research are posed in such a way as to allow the respondent free expression.

Validity   The ability of a data collecting method or instrument to measure what it is supposed to measure.

Variable   Any characteristic, quality or attribute that varies, can be observed and can be measured.

Index